"An amazing piece of work. It made me smile and cry at the same time and I really feel every woman on the planet needs to read it."

Dr Louise Newson

"A genuine triumph over adversity; what you have created is invaluable. If you have a vagina, know or love somebody with a vagina, you need to read this book."

Diane Danzebrink, The Menopause Counsellor

"I love the book and already have patients and friends in mind that I can recommend it to. Reading Jane's story has given me a greater insight into the huge effects that vaginal atrophy has on a woman's life."

Fiona Mitchell, Women's Health Physiotherapist

"This is a very brave and frank description of one woman's plight against the symptoms of vaginal atrophy that is both informative and educational. I would recommend it to everyone."

Amanda Tozer, Consultant Gynaecologist

"Absolutely love it! Such an honest and informative read, smashing the taboo surrounding the conversation about our vaginas."

Sam Evans, Sexual Health Expert

"This book is refreshingly candid and one of a kind.

"As you read it, you will find yourself laughing out loud at the authors humour. She takes you on a journey of vaginal awareness; giving both factual information and sharing her painful, personal journey with vaginal atrophy.

"The author's writing style is conversational and easy to read; to the extent that you feel like you are sitting in the kitchen with her, having a chat over coffee. It seems to me that the main motivations of the book are: to promote vaginal and vulval health; to empower women to seek help; to offer encouragement, information and resources to fellow sufferers. The book raises questions and challenges the boundaries of your comfort zones.

"This extraordinary, outstanding book is well worth a read. It is the sort of book that you will buy extra copies of, to give it to your daughters, your sisters and your friends."

Julie Bennett, Educational Author

Me and My Menopausal Vagina

Living with Vaginal Atrophy

Jane Lewis

Published by

PAL Books

First published in Great Britain in 2018 by PAL Books

© Jane Lewis

First Edition

ISBN (print): 978-1-9164467-0-0
ISBN (kindle): 978-1-9164467-1-7
ISBN (ePub): 978-1-9164467-2-4

DISCLAIMER

A CIP catalogue record for this book is available from the British Library.

This book can be ordered from:
ypdbooks.com
mymenopausalvagina.co.uk
mymenopausalvagina.com
Amazon Books
Waterstones

Written by Penny Lewis (Jane's daughter)

Cover Design image(s) used under license from InkDrop/shutterstock.com

Illustrations by studiostunner.com

Page Layout / Typesetting: Chris Moore

This book is dedicated to you.
I hope that you find some comfort between
both these pages and your legs!

A Little Note Before Reading

Let's quickly clear something up: perimenopause, meno-pause and post-menopause are not the same thing.

Perimenopause refers to the period of time it takes for your body to change from a woman who can reproduce to a woman who can't. This transition period can last many years and is usually where most women experience their symptoms: night sweats, hot flushes, mood swings, forgetful-ness, vaginal atrophy. If you're of menopausal age but are still having periods, however irregular, you're in perimenopause.

Once you've not had a period for an entire year, you can then say you're menopausal. Despite our regular misuse of the word, menopause actually refers only to a particular day: day 365 of not having a period.

Everything after that event refers to post-menopause.

For the purposes of this book however, I've used the more widely accepted term menopause to act as a catch-all for peri-menopause and post-menopause. This is because in some places the writing became a bit confusing and the meaning was lost. Please be aware therefore that this interchange of menopause, perimenopause and post-menopause was a conscious decision for ease of reading and understanding.

Also, as I will be discussing my experiences of living with vaginal atrophy, let's just be clear about its meaning. Vaginal atrophy refers to the drying, shrinking, thinning and inflammation of the vaginal walls and vulva area. This is as a result of low oestrogen levels in the body which are especially low during menopause. As it sounds, vaginal atrophy is pretty horrific and can cause a lot of pain and discomfort, not just when having sex, but all the time. Some women may also experience really awful urinary symptoms, including constant and seemingly incurable urinary tract infections (UTIs). Even though the term was rebranded Genitourinary Syndrome of Menopause, many women still refer to it as vaginal atrophy or VA and so that is what I'll be using throughout the book.

Let's begin.

How to Find Your Way Around

Preface

Vagina.

There, I've said it. Let's get the meet-and-greet out the way and get stuck right in – so to speak.

Ladies, before we begin I think it's important to set a few things straight. We do not have front bottoms, or foofs, lady gardens, or minis. Nor do we have clunges, or lady bits, fannies or 'down theres' and we most *certainly* do not have twats!

No, ladies, we have vaginas and vulvas, and they are *not* dirty words.

For too long we have failed to really *accept* our vaginas: adopting instead the *out of sight, out of mind* mentality that has led to a culture of secrecy and shame. Unlike our male counterparts who can whip out theirs willy-nilly, our genitals are hidden within us, and that can often mean that our suffering of it is too.

We have been made to think that our vaginas and vulvas are something to be ashamed of, or that need to be groomed and pruned, or plucked and shaved for another's benefit. Ladies, we pluck *turkeys*, groom *dogs* and prune *hedges* – we need to start reclaiming our genitals as our own and start to understand them properly.

And we *especially* need to start talking about our vulvas and vaginas as they start to age: what to expect, what to do and who to see. Society has somehow sanitised the menopausal woman; hot flushes and hysteria seem to be the current 'funny' stereotype. Cartoons are made of women standing naked in front of a fridge to cool herself down, or of a husband tip-toeing carefully around his angry hormonal wife, who no doubt has crazy frizzy hair and bright red cheeks. The menopausal woman is known to be hot, forgetful and a bit manic; an easy type-cast.

But what happens when we cool the flushes, or level the hormones and start to deal with some of the other devastating, not so PG-friendly symptoms: the vaginal dryness, the burning vulva, the suicidal depression? Why doesn't that form part of the stock character that a menopausal woman is cast as? It is simply unacceptable that *vaginal atrophy* isn't part of our general vocabulary of the ageing woman; just because it is hidden, does not mean it should be kept a secret.

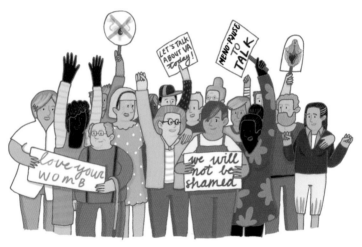

And so I'd like to tell you about my own experiences so that you don't feel alone, isolated, or ashamed. In writing this book, I hope to dispel the shame and secrecy of vaginal dryness and atrophy and hope to give you the courage to start a dialogue with your friends, family and colleagues, so that you can start sharing your troubles and find help together. But although this book is written from my point of view as a woman with vaginal atrophy at menopause, I believe it should be a must-read for young girls too. If you can learn about good vaginal health when you're young, you'll be better equipped to deal with some of the potential effects of ageing. If you've never heard of the Bartholin glands, introitus, vestibule or perineum and still couldn't confidently label all the bits on your genitals, I think this book will help you. Whether you've had sex for the first time, have just given birth, have survived vulval cancer but are left with unimaginable vaginal dryness, are being driven mad by pudendal neuralgia, have pelvic floor disfunction (PFD), painful bladder syndrome (PBS) or vulvodynia, this book is for you.

But before I open up about my experience, I need you to know that I am not an expert. I am not a doctor or a nurse and I have no medical qualifications whatsoever. I didn't go to university to study medicine or biology.

In fact, I didn't go to university at all.

But what I have done is birth three tear-jerkingly big babies, weep my way through the same number of episiotomies and survive a few pretty horrendous years of perimenopause – bracing myself for the years ahead. I'd even go as far to say I've become something of a vagina whizz over the last seven years – a strange triumph, I know.

From the knowledge I've acquired and the willingness to talk openly about vaginal atrophy (VA) and vulva issues, I've become something of a signpost and agony aunt for suffering women: directing them where to go, what to do and who to turn to. I've appeared on TV, on the radio and in a magazine, attended lectures, conferences and appointments with specialists and have been asked to try and test products that claim to help VA. Some doctors, therapists and women's health physiotherapists are now even recommending their patients to get in touch with me so that I can give advice or guidance on how best to manage their symptoms – from one sufferer to the other. I've picked up the phone and replied to thousands of messages from many desperate women all over the world and many have claimed that I've literally saved their lives – if not, at least, their vaginas! Through my journey and through the women I've met along the way, I've come to realise that we *can* survive the challenges yet to come, that we can strive to understand what our bodies are going through and that, in turn, we can learn to, if not love, then at least *accept* our vaginas.

And so, with a deep breath, I'd like to introduce you to someone who, despite my choice or better judgement, has become very important in my life. She is 52 years old, has rather unruly hair and has a face like a smacked bottom. She never does what I tell her to, and goes hot and cold on me all the time. Living with her has become something of a nightmare. In truth, she's a bit of a bitch.

So, ladies and gentlemen, please be nice.

Welcome, to my vagina.

CHAPTER 1

Who Am I?

Hello.

I'm Jane and, like my vagina, I'm 52 years old. I live with my husband of 34 years, have three grown up daughters, a granddaughter, and two dogs: Bertie and Bonnie.

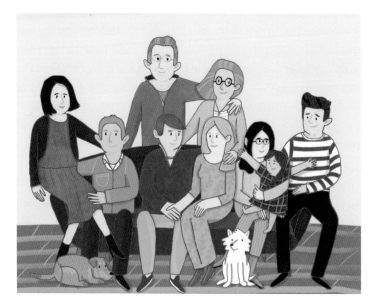

I used to live a really active life: horse-riding, swimming, walking, cycling. Sitting down for hours at a time wouldn't even cross my mind as being a problem; I could go to the cinema, sit at a restaurant and go on long car journeys like anyone else.

I'm a florist by trade and had my own floristry business, creating floral arrangements for an award-winning hotel. I could stand for hours putting together the bouquets, table arrangements and button holes for the never ending merry-go-round of brides (and bridezillas!) and found it no bother at all lifting the heavy flower boxes and watering cans in and out of the car.

I was happy.

Of course, like everyone else I had my own worries in life, but with my three chicks having flown the nest and a freshly hatched one chirping away, I was really enjoying the dizzying chaos of being a grandma for the first time. I was looking forward to watching my granddaughter grow up and go stomping in puddles like I used to with my own girls. I was fit and kept a little horse on a scrap of land in the neighbouring village, imagining that one day I'd go there with my granddaughter and we'd play ponies together. I'd have her on my shoulders, swing her by the arm and bounce her on my knee when we got back home.

But then something changed.

I'm not quite sure the exact moment when things went so drastically downhill, but I do remember one day being at the cinema and suddenly realising that I couldn't sit down. After only 20 minutes, I took myself to the back of the theatre and stood alone, swaying from side to side try-ing to calm the burning. I haven't been able to sit through a film since.

If I look back now, I can see that there were already little signs that something was wrong when I was around 45: finding underwear uncomfortable, feeling suddenly very aware of my vulva, getting vaginal ache after a long day standing as a florist. As strange as it now sounds to me,

I didn't think anything of it – just getting on with my day, going commando when my vulva felt sensitive and taking some painkillers if I got sore.

Fast-forward 7 years and I no longer work, have visited an uncountable number of medical health professionals (many are experts in their field), wept my way around almost every local park, and had my vagina lasered like a Star Wars lightsaber. Though I'm now much better than I was at the start of my journey, there is still a long road ahead.

I've learnt that, like the greys on my head and the wrinkles on my face, my vulva and vagina age as well and that sometimes the results can be grim.

But how grim?

Well, I have or have had stabbing pains in my vagina, burning in my vulva, constant soreness, micro-cuts on my perineum, thinning skin that leads to splitting (including from my episiotomies), seemingly never-ending urinary tract infections (UTIs), itching, ulcers, a painful clitoris, and very very sensitive skin. My pubes starting shedding like a sheep in the spring, wearing *any* knickers or trousers was excruciating and sex? Ha! Forget it. That ship has sailed.

I've been to counsellors, doctors, nutritionists, physiotherapists, gynaecologists, vulva-dermatologists, pain specialists, uro-gynaecologists, sexual health specialists and medical herbalists.

I've had acupuncture, hypnotherapy, reiki, spiritual healing, massages, reflexology and CBT.

I've tried and applied almost every cream, lubricant and moisturiser there is, spending literally thousands of pounds that I don't have on trying to find 'a cure'. Having never had a facial in my life or worn makeup or moisturised, I now

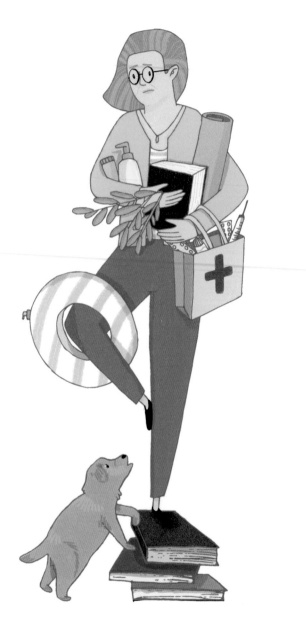

have a strict 'vacial' routine where I foof my vagina and vulva and pamper to its every whim twice a day. If the local beauty salon started doing vacials, I have no doubt I would be their best customer!

I've been given anti-depressants, antibiotics, weird and wonderful lotions and potions from varying 'specialists', vitamins, health supplements and finally, after wading through a quagmire of bureaucratic, misinformed and unnecessarily confusing nonsense, HRT. We'll return to this later.

But as well as the physical pain, I've also suffered mentally: panic attacks, anxiety, confusion and severe depression, at times even considering suicide.

One of the hardest things I found when I first started experiencing vaginal problems was the inability to discuss what I was going through openly with friends and family. It's a very isolating feeling when you suffer from a condition or from pain in a 'private' area; unlike your back or a more 'socially acceptable' ailment, telling every Tom, Dick and Harry about your itching, sore, broken vagina doesn't seem to get you many friends. In fact, in my experience it could mean losing some of them.

And so, despite being totally computer-illiterate, I set up an online support group for 'women like me' who might need a safe-place to discuss their worries and woes.

The support group started off as a way to feed my own curiosity – *was I the only one like this?* – and now serves as a support for hundreds of women from all over the world. I believe there are many thousands more who would benefit from being part of such a community, so they can see that they are not alone and receive support and advice from other women going through something similar.

Perhaps you are one of these women?

Every day I receive, and personally vet, requests from women who have – to a lesser or greater degree – something wrong with their vagina or vulva. It might be the 23 year old who has just started experiencing dryness when she has sex, or the 73 year old who can't bear to keep her 'shameful secret' a secret any longer. The group acts as a virtual living room where women can chat about their various problems and seek to help each other through it. Sometimes the advice given on these pages is more insightful than the thousands of pounds spent desperately at private medical centres; sometimes too the non-judgement and frank discussion is enough to keep a woman from killing herself.

To some, this may sound all too familiar and to others it may seem unimaginable or perhaps even melodramatic. To those who can understand this physical and mental torment, I reach out to you across the page and say "I get it, I'm sorry, and, you're strong". Please don't feel alone. You are not.

To those who may find these words dramatic, I am genuinely pleased for you that you have been spared this awful affliction; I would not wish this upon my enemy. But I'd also ask you to be kind, and to not judge these emotions. Until we experience something ourselves, it is often difficult to really understand what it is like or how we would handle a similar situation. Some of the saddest moments in life are when we share a suffering with someone we trust and we learn that they are not strong enough or comfortable enough to hear it or that, because of their own experiences, they are unable to listen non-judgmentally and compassionately.

Make sure *you* listen.

Let's not belittle our sisters just because you got through menopause relatively unharmed; let's not shut them out because you feel uncomfortable talking about vaginal

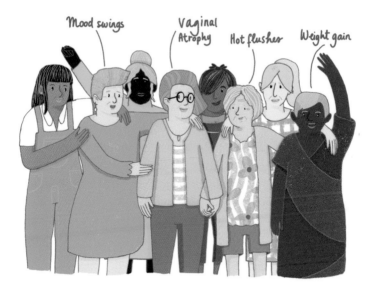

dryness; let's be here, ready to talk to each other and support each other in whatever way we may need.

If you're a man reading this, welcome! We're very pleased to have you here. This isn't a woman's problem, it's a societal problem and we need to make sure we're ridding the shame of it so that better treatment can be found. So, please share this book with your friends, mothers, daughters, sons, husbands, wives, partners, neighbours, and most definitely, your doctor.

The first step, though, is in knowing your vagina.

CHAPTER 2

This is Your Vagina

First things first: you need to be clear about what and where your vagina actually is. This might sound rather silly as, after all, it is *that thing down there*. Yet surprisingly, it was only during a conversation with my daughter whilst writing this book that I realised that even within my own home, there wasn't a proper understanding of it.

So, let's take a peek.

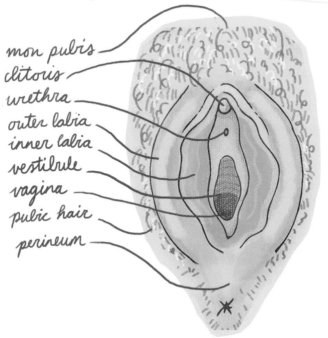

mon pubis
clitoris
urethra
outer labia
inner labia
vestibule
vagina
pubic hair
perineum

Unless you're reading this on a train, a bus, or in a doctor's surgery, please go grab yourself a mirror or shimmy up to a full-length one and get ready to be enlightened.

But a word of warning: if any of what you're about to read is totally new to you, I'd suggest coming back to this chapter a couple of times to make sure it all sinks in. And please do go off and do your own research – our bodies are pretty incredible machines and taking the time to understand exactly how and why they work will help us no end when they inevitably start to seize up a bit.

Ready?

Pubic hair

OK, so when you're standing naked in front of the mirror with your legs closed, you can see your *mons pubis*, or *pubic hair* as you probably call it.

This is not your vagina.

If, like me, you're *organic* in your approach to hair maintenance, this'll likely be covered in enough hair to make the Amazon rainforest look sparse. Please be aware though that depending on individual body differences or where you are in your menopause journey, your pubic hair may have seriously reduced in thickness or perhaps even died out entirely. This is likely to be as a result of very low levels of oestrogen in your body and shouldn't alone be a reason to worry – but of course head to your doctor if you'd like to have some peace of mind. At one point my public hair was so grey and thinning, not even a comb-over would have made it look normal! It wasn't until I started rebalancing my hormones that it began to grow back. I am pleased to say that once again I have the pleasure of watching my locks of greying

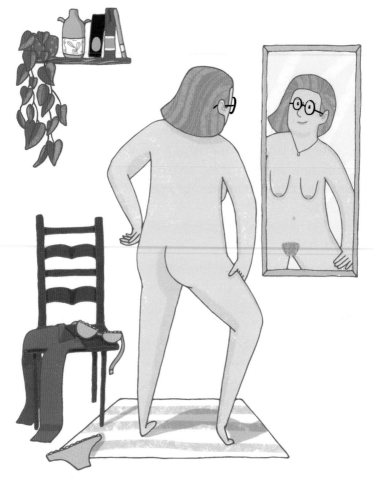

pubes hang desperately out the sides of my Bridget Jones' knickers, like spiders fleeing a scooping mug. Alas!

Vulva

Now, if you open your legs without yet prodding around, what you see is your *vulva* – the collective name for your *external* genitals. The vulva includes your outer and inner labia, clitoris, urethra and vestibule. Again, this isn't your vagina because your vagina is hidden. The likelihood is that you've been calling this your vagina all your life; you're wrong. It would be the same as calling your lips and mouth your throat; the throat is on the inside and your lips are what can be seen on the outside. Your vulva is like your lips, and your vagina is like your throat.

Why is this important?

Well, it's important we know what we're talking about if we're trying to explain a pain. It's a strange thing that we're so unaware of a vital part of our bodies: the part that births human life, maintains its own ecosystem, feels good during sex. Without knowing exactly what we're talking about, we're not able to properly direct a medical professional to *where* it's hurting when something feels wrong. "*My vagina is painful*" is simply too vague a term: is it the vestibule, the clitoris, the perineum, the labia? You wouldn't go to a doctor and say your 'face' hurts: you'd say your *ear*, or *eye*, or *nose*. We must do the same with our genitalia to ensure we receive the proper diagnosis and treatment.

OK, so your legs are open, you can see your vulva – let's look at the individual parts contained within it.

Outer labia

The larger spongey area that looks a bit like a mini hotdog bun is the *outer labia* or *labia majora*. Like the pubic hair, the outer labia acts as another barrier to protect the vagina from any external threats – like when rugby players wear gum-shields to protect their teeth. Though, in this instance, (unfortunately/thank God), you're unlikely to have the whole rugby team hurtling themselves towards your vagina!

For me, the skin around my vulva has been one of my biggest problem areas and was where I first started to experience symptoms: insatiable itching, soreness when I was sitting down, hypersensitivity when I was wearing knickers. By this stage, sex had become quite painful and I was noticing that I'd get up and go to the toilet multiple times a night. Strangely too, I also had severe itching all over the rest of my body, particularly on my shins and around my face, ears and eyes. It's only now that I realise this was due to my oestrogen levels dropping and my body not being able to handle it. I guess I was almost going into a state of withdrawal. Officially, this crazy itching which felt like ants were crawling under my skin, is known as *formication* and is due to our bodies not being able to produce oils or moisture anymore from not having enough oestrogen. If you're experiencing this manic itching, head to your doctor to discuss your treatment options because it's *awful* and you shouldn't have to put up with it.

Like a grape to a raisin, with age the plumpness of your whole body and therefore your outer labia will also reduce, potentially leaving it more sensitive or painful. We'll explore different treatments, medications and products for these symptoms later on.

Inner labia

Depending on how Mother Nature designed you, your *inner labia* or *labia minora* may, like your belly-button, be an outie or an innie. This means that the inner labia may or may not be visible when your legs are closed, perhaps even poking out through the outer labia lips. Ladies, aesthetically, it does not matter which one you have. The amount of girls I hear about who are having a labiaplasty *purely* because they *don't like the way their labias look* or are worried they '*aren't normal*' is shocking. Where are they getting these ideas from? Since when are labias *supposed* to look pretty?

I'm sure there's more than one contributing factor to this trend but I'd bet a small sum that social media and the porn industry have had some hand in it: putting pressure on our girls to look a certain way, or live up to unrealistic images. It was for that reason that I consciously walked around the house naked when my girls were growing up; I wanted them to see what a *real* woman's body looked like, with all the stretch marks, cellulite and doughy tummy hanging out.

I needed them to know that the images they saw in magazines weren't really normal, even though that's how the industry wanted you to feel. It would be like us looking through a gardening magazine and feeling suddenly ashamed that our dying grass patch wasn't up to Chelsea standards, or feeling unworthy that our pastry didn't rise as well as Delia's. Of course, there are always some girls or women who *need* to have such surgeries for medical reasons and I hope that they are being adequately educated to ensure they can go into menopause knowing what to look out for and what to do if they start experiencing any problems.

Like the outer, the *inner labia's* job is also to protect your vagina from infection, acting almost like curtains, with the grand opening being your vagina. Over the surface of the inner labia are lots of miniscule glands whose job it is to lubricate the area, like a mechanic with a bit of WD-40®. When menopause hits, this mechanic basically sods off and leaves you choking on the driveway like an engine without oil; our job is to become our own mechanic and find other ways to lubricate our vaginas and vulvas. We'll look into these a bit later.

However, it's important you know that you might not actually *have* any inner labia left – with it having reduced in size so much that you can barely even see it. This reduction in both size and plumpness is most likely as a result of chronically low oestrogen levels and, unfortunately, is pretty common among menopausal women. You might also find that it's much drier than it used to be and may even stick together like the pages of a wet book. By trying the different products and treatment methods we explore later, there's a good chance you'll be able to bring back some moisture and ease the discomfort. So if you're sitting with your legs spread-eagled and are searching for your inner labia like a squirrel digging for nuts in the winter, do not panic yet. There are many reasons why it may have gone AWOL *but* a good rule of thumb is: If it shocks, go to the docs!

My friend, for example, after hearing about the problems *I* was having with my vulvovaginal area, decided to take a look at herself in the mirror for the first time ever and found nothing at all. But by *nothing* I don't mean she found nothing *wrong*: there was literally no labia left. It had shrivelled up completely and was barely visible. For her, she later found out that she was suffering from *lichen sclerosus*, but had she not been almost forced to take a peek, she could potentially have left the condition untreated and developed something much more serious.

But even if you *do* still have your labia minora, please be aware that it's likely to shrink in size, lose its sponginess and become quite thin and frail. These are not things to be worried about, they are just to be aware of, so that you can start treating it as soon as you notice it's starting to struggle. I left mine too late. For me, this area became so painful I could no longer sit down, wear trousers or even underwear; it felt like I was literally sitting on a wasp nest which no position seemed to ease. I tried creams, moisturisers, ointments and pills but in the end, it was a combination of lots of things together that was my salvation: HRT, local oestrogen, laser treatment, women's health physiotherapy and the daily application of different products. We'll have a look at all of these in a moment.

So ladies, *please* have a look at yourself. It's not dirty, it's not weird, and it might just save your life.

Clitoris

Do you all know where your clitoris is? It looks a bit like the jibbly-bits on a rooster's head and can be found just below where the inner labia meet. As you or your partner might have already found out, this is a very sensitive area which can help women reach climax if it's stimulated in a pleasurable way. Interestingly, the clitoris isn't just the wibbly bit you can see, it also branches off like a wish-bone into your genitalia and is about 3 inches in length. Imagine it being like a jellyfish in the ocean: although the bit above the water is what *we* can see, there are also tentacles (in our case, two) anchoring it below. Depending on your body, some women have clitoral and some women have vaginal orgasms during sex so it's really worth getting to know your body to understand what you like and what you don't. And did you know that the clitoris has around 8000 nerve endings compared to the penis, which has around only half of that? Cool, hey? Whilst this can be great, it also explains why some women can experience so much pain when their clitoris becomes hypersensitive.

Like a wizard's robe, the clitoris has a hood over it, aptly named the *clitoral hood*, which should slide-n-glide nicely, protecting the clitoral gland. But, with menopause, this too can atrophy, exposing the extremely sensitive gland below.

For a while, I even suffered from something called *permanent genital arousal disorder (PGAD)* which meant the clitoral gland was permanently sensitised from its lack of protection – like a root exposed on your tooth. This, despite what some may think, was absolutely awful and led me into serious depression and suicidal thoughts. The embarrassment and shame I felt was doubly heavy, as even those who I turned to for help, medically and non-medically, seemed to wince and cower when I brought it up.

In our society, talking about genitalia and sex seems to be viewed despairingly and even I would have seen it as a taboo subject had it not literally taken over my life. But because I felt so dirty and helpless with PGAD, I was not able to get the help I ultimately needed until much later down the line when I was brave/desperate enough to speak out. Until we're prepared to sit in our GP's room and look the doctor in the eye without flinching, we're never going to change the current stigma attached to menopause and women's health.

Urethra

Underneath your clitoris is your urethra; *this* is where you wee from. I've recently chatted with a 60 year old who thought all her life that she wee'd out of her vagina: you don't. Don't feel silly if you thought this too, I think it's very common.

During menopause, UTIs become very common due to the fact that the urethra and a section of the bladder called the *trigone area* are very oestrogen dependent; when they no longer have the oestrogen they need, they become more prone to infection. This is probably a good place to pause for a moment to consider the disastrous design of our genitals. Who, in their right mind, would build a theme park next to a sewage works? Think about how the same applies to us…

I've heard from literally thousands of women on my support groups who've got caught up in a yo-yo of short-term low-dose antibiotics, prescribed by doctors, in an attempt to rid themselves of the infection. Don't let this be you; the infection will only come back to haunt you if you don't treat it properly, like that weed that keeps coming back because you haven't pulled it out by the roots. Have a proper dialogue with your doctor about the most appropriate treatment for *you* and take the time to understand what you're taking. Luckily, my doctor has been fabulous and prescribed me local oestrogen and HRT which stopped the yo-yo and eradicated most of the UTI symptoms: such as burning, stinging, leaking, and a desperate need to *Go Now*. Although my bladder is in no way perfect, the discomfort is manageable and has reduced my nightly pee-sessions to one. Perhaps this is something you could discuss with your doctor too.

Women who are breastfeeding or who've recently had a baby may be showing symptoms of UTIs and vaginal atrophy. This is because they're also lacking oestrogen. It might be worth just asking your friend/relative whether they're OK 'down there' or whether they need to be prescribed local oestrogen for the short term until they finish breast-feeding. In any event, if *my* daughter's had episiotomy scars, I'd recommend for them to go to their GP to discuss whether they should rub local oestrogen into them twice daily to help the healing process.

Vestibule

OK, so the outer and inner labia are open – what you can now see is your *vestibule*. If we were at the theatre, the labia flaps would be like the stage *curtains*, the vestibule would be the *stage* and the vagina would be *backstage* (in the wings, and deep in the darkness).

During our reproductive years, something called the *Bartholin glands* (which sit just inside the vagina at 5 and 7 o'clock) produce mucus to lubricate the vulva for sex and everyday living. Think back to the mechanic with the WD-40®. This is why our vulva and vagina should hopefully not cause us too much jip when we're younger; our bread, as it were, is well and truly buttered. However, skip forward to menopause and our vagina becomes like a dry piece of wholemeal bread that even the birds would struggle to swallow.

For me, the discomfort from my vestibule felt like a shoe was rubbing a blister all day, and there was no option to remove it. When moisturised twice a day however, the pain reduced; but even now with HRT and local oestrogen, I'm still very aware of the soreness between my legs. Some vulva-dermatologists even suggest moisturising your vulva twice daily from 40 years onwards, after all, if our skin on our face wrinkles, so too does the skin down below. I strongly believe that if I'd been educated earlier and had started some of these moisturising treatments in my early 40s, then I may have warded off some of my more severe symptoms.

If you've had children, your vestibule might look a bit Frankenstein-esque with episiotomies scaring the surface. Remember that when your skin starts to shrivel and tighten, so too will your scars, so keep an eye on them if they become painful. Because I've had three 9lb+ babies, my vestibule loosely resembles a shot pigeon: where you know what you're supposed to be looking at but somehow you struggle to make out the specifics. Don't worry if it looks more Picasso than Da Vinci down there; just be aware that if it becomes sore, there might be something you can do to help it.

In between the Bartholin glands is the *introitus* which is basically the entrance into the vagina. This is where a lot of women experience pain during sex, where there may be so much dryness and thinning skin that it can literally split open.

For me, this is a problem even today.

Every time I wee, the acid from the urine burns the skin and causes me a lot of discomfort, so it's very important that I keep to my strict moisturising 'vacial' routine and am careful when I wipe myself – which is more of a dab than a sweep. I know of many women who take a bottle of water into the toilet with them to rinse themselves after each wee and for them it seems to be helping, so it might be something you could consider if you're experiencing similar problems. Just make sure you don't get your Coca Cola mixed up with your Evian, otherwise you might be in trouble.

Now we're through the introitus, you have finally arrived at your destination: your vagina.

Vagina

Let's have a look around.

In our younger days, our vaginas were structured with something called *rugae* which are very similar to pleats of a curtain or the bellows of an accordion: all rouched up and ready to expand when necessary to let the penis in and the baby out. In other words, the rugae allows the vagina to stretch open and lengthen and then retract again to minimise tearing. The only time we don't have rugae is when we're prepubescent and then menopausal. To get an idea about what these rugae are like, put your tongue on the roof of your mouth towards your front teeth; can you feel the bumpy ridges? That's basically what your rugae are like in your vagina (but without the teeth!). Once these pleats have smoothed out, the vagina becomes shorter, tighter and is more at risk of tearing from intercourse and even, in some cases, sticking together. That's why learning about what you can do to take care of your genitals is really important.

At the top of your vagina is your cervix, the neck of the womb. Without getting too medical, the cervix produces mucus which goes down into the vagina to keep everything lubricated and healthy, and then eventually onto your lovely lace knickers. However, with menopause this mucus dries up.

I first noticed this when I was around 40 years old; I realised I hadn't had discharge in my knickers for a while. But then, after a few years, the discharge came back resembling in its appearance, milk. Unlike our younger days when the discharge should be more like egg whites, mine had now changed. On the surface, this may not feel like vaginal dryness as, after all, you are *wet* rather than dry, but don't be fooled. Many women think this is thrush rather than vaginal atrophy and so go about self-treating with over-the-counter products which, over time, may actually make the problem worse. What you actually need is our friend, local oestrogen, and we'll look at that in more detail later.

If, during sex, you notice any bleeding you *must* go to see your GP to ensure you have all necessary investigations. This bleeding is likely to be coming from your vaginal walls and may be as a result of the onset of vaginal atrophy or other, unlikely but potentially serious conditions. Relying solely on social media or forums for a diagnosis isn't a good idea as it is likely that no one, including myself, is medically trained to give advice that could potentially be very serious.

So ladies, *this* is your vagina, and *this* is why you need to know your vulva from your vestibule and your clitoris from your urethra. Just flick back through the last few pages to see how many parts we've looked at (and that therefore may be causing you pain) and none of that was your vagina. See how important it is to know your anatomy? Only then will you be able to tell your doctor exactly where it's hurting, and only then will they be able to properly help you.

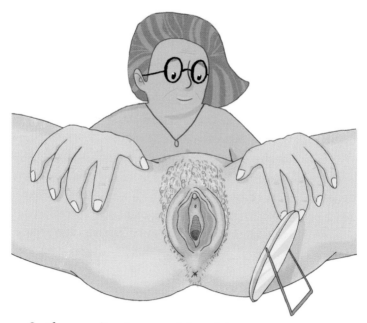

So if you can't point to each bit of this picture and explain what it's called and what it does, have another read of the chapter. Try to apply it to your own symptoms and start to be more specific about where your pain is coming from.

CHAPTER 3

Vaginal Atrophy

Never mind the symptoms, the name itself is depressing enough. Why couldn't it be called something else? Something less, I don't know, *vaginal*. It just feels so clinical and graphic and sterile – no wonder no-one wants to talk about it! If only we could be referring to our *mature* vaginas, instead – that would feel better, wouldn't it? We'd stop viewing them as burdens and instead see them like those wise old tribeswomen who have seen a lot of things and now walk nonchalantly around with a stick and an air of mystique and knowledge. Our mature, aged vaginas would tell all the younger, less experienced vaginas about the ways of the world and would read them stories of myth and legend and teach them how things used to be. Or perhaps, we could claim *vintage* as our own? It seems to have gone down pretty well for wine and cheese so I see no real barrier to adding a third item to that category. The vintage vagina. I like it. But *vaginal atrophy*? Eurgh! The *wasting away* of our vaginas. Gross! And even the 2014 name change to *Genitourinary Syndrome of Menopause* doesn't seem to have helped much: I mean, how many of us can even actually pronounce it?

I wish I had been aware of what to expect. Though it wouldn't have necessarily changed anything, it would have made me feel better prepared to deal with the horrors of vaginal atrophy (VA). I would have known that the burning and the soreness was due to my ageing vagina and that there might be something more I could do to help myself out: some people to go to, some products to try. I might even have started thinking about appropriate treatments earlier than I eventually did, spending so much of those early days getting acquainted with the condition and trying to figure out what it was I was actually dealing with.

So, if you're new to VA, or if you've grappled with it for a while but are still chasing your tail about what to do, perhaps I can signpost you in some of the directions that worked for me? Over the next couple of chapters, I briefly mention the most prominent symptoms that have negatively affected my life, and discuss who I went to in order to sort it out and how I've managed to get on top of it.

Tips

"And it burns, burns, burns, the ring of fire, the ring of fire..."

Never before had I felt closer to Johnny Cash than when I first started getting vaginal problems. I'm sure it wasn't part of his creative process to think about the ageing vaginas of menopausal women, but he does seem to have some alarmingly accurate insight!

Who knew it could *burn, burn, burn* so much?

Ice packs, heat packs, frozen tins and vegetables all went between my legs in an attempt to calm the flame, and my day revolved around freezing different food items and kitchenware to find the best results. In the early days of my atrophy, I remember reading on a blog somewhere that frozen food cans remained cool for up to 10 hours and that they could be used to keep a picnic chilled throughout the day. Brilliant, I thought! If it works for scotch eggs, it'll do nicely for my vagina. And so, one day, when my son-in-law was trying to make beans on toast but couldn't find the tins, I had to explain to him why exactly they were now frozen and therefore out of action…

The things we do, eh?

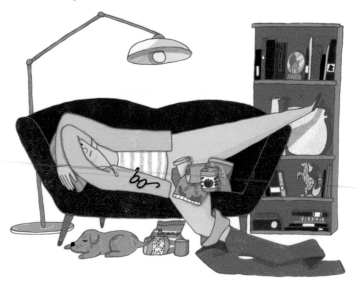

But you know what? It helped! As much as the picture of me lying on the sofa with a tin of frozen baked beans wedged between my thighs couldn't exactly be described as a high point in my life, the temporary relief from the burning did give me back some normality to my day. For a few hours, the pain dulled into a background ache and I could focus on something else for a bit. Even if that 'something' was further research on how to heal a broken vagina.

Ironically too, heat also seemed to help – especially on my bladder area – and so I'd plug myself into a heat-pad I bought cheaply online and would both freeze and bake throughout the day. A bit like warm apple crumble with ice-cream.

A problem I found, though, was that I seemed to have become very sensitive to *anything* touching my vulva area, including knickers and trousers. For many months I found it unbearable to wear underwear or jeans, or indeed anything too tight around my skin, leaving me with little else but long skirts and the natural air on my bottom half (and praying to high heaven that a gust of wind wouldn't suddenly expose me to a passerby). I remember my daughter telling me one day that my three year old granddaughter had taken great delight in telling her nursery that "Grandma doesn't wear knickers anymore". True I guess.

Though I can now wear underwear again, if you're suffering from vaginal burning and need immediate relief, I'd suggest having a go with frozen cans and heat pads: they're cheap and easy to do at home. But obviously, ladies, although we want to cool down the burning we don't want frostbite, so please make sure you're wrapping things up in a cloth or a towel. I'd usually have about five different food cans on rotation that I'd freeze overnight ready to be used for the next morning, and then another set that I could take to bed with me. I even know of ladies who have taken a heat or a cool pad into work to sit on and have just told their colleagues they had back ache – what their colleagues didn't know however was that earlier that morning they also had a chilled dilator stuffed up their vagina as well!

But though this method might offer you some respite from the unbearable burning, realistically, boiling and freezing your genitals probably isn't the answer and ultimately our aim is to find a longer term solution.

Though I hope that you've already gone to your doctor to discuss your VA, and that they've been able to signpost you in some useful directions, there are a few things that I didn't even know existed at the beginning of my journey. For example, it might be that a couple of trips to your women's health physiotherapist does the trick and helps your VA, or that laser treatment is your saving grace, or HRT, or local oestrogen, or simply a change in lifestyle. We all know that being fit and healthy, though not always fun, can have a powerful positive impact on our bodies; some women have noticed a real change in their symptoms simply through ditching the booze and sugar and taking up yoga and spinach instead. A trip therefore to a nutritionist might work wonders for you. Or it might not. What is important is that you *try* different methods; invest time and energy in yourself to make sure you're doing whatever you can to maximise your quality of life and lower your pain. Don't give up.

Let's look at some of these options in a bit more detail to see if there's anything that might help you.

CHAPTER 4

Treatments

Local oestrogen

The first time you go to the doctor discussing your VA, you might be offered one of two things: thrush cream or local oestrogen. If you're offered thrush cream and don't have thrush, don't use it. This might sound very obvious but I've heard of a staggering number of women who are having their VA misdiagnosed as thrush that can be supposedly cured by a short application of thrush cream. Be careful. If you continue to apply thrush cream to your VA, you're likely to make the matter much, much worse, so please ask your doctor how they know that it's thrush rather than VA.

If you're offered oestrogen, you might be prescribed only a very short course of *local* oestrogen – *locally* just meaning that you apply it straight onto and into your vulvovaginal area. As we'll see in more detail in Chapter 5, oestrogen is integral to the proper functioning of our bodies and in the case of VA it helps to improve vaginal lubrication. Basically, by applying local oestrogen you're bringing back the mechanic with the WD-40® we spoke about in Chapter 3 who is oiling your hinges and preventing you from getting stuck again. It also helps to calm the burning by lowering the pH level of your vagina, thickening up the body's tissue (known as the *epithelium*), and increasing blood flow to your vulva and vagina – giving you back a spongier, fuller area that you had when you were younger. This is important because it helps to keep the area nice and cushioned, protected and hydrated which in turn helps to reduce associated problems from atrophy. Who knew we would one day be longing for our spongey vulvas?

Though local oestrogen can be brilliant, it isn't *so* brilliant that it can necessarily cure you from one application. I mean, if we just doused a wilting plant with a tonne of water but never watered it again, we probably wouldn't expect it to live for all that long. The same goes for our vaginas and vulvas. Like a plant, we need to help it out by providing it with the essential nutrients all year round, that it cannot otherwise get from the soil. And yet, of the hundreds of women on my online support group, an alarming number of them seem to be prescribed very short-term treatments that promise to *fix'em up good an' proper* from one go. This worries me on several levels.

First of all, I just can't see how it can be the case that an area of your body that has been so desperately deprived of oestrogen and other essential hormones can suddenly have gotten all it needs forevermore from a short course of topical treatment. It would be like giving a young woman three contraceptive pills and telling her that it'd probably last the year. Or applying sunscreen only once and then expecting your skin not to burn.

There seems to be an almost embedded fear or misunderstanding around oestrogen which is leaving women being refused the treatment they so desperately need. It should be absolute basic knowledge that local oestrogen is *safe* for most women; in fact, the amount of oestrogen you're getting from the treatment is so low that a *year's* supply of local oestrogen is the equivalent to taking only *one tablet* of the lowest dose of HRT. *One tablet for a whole year's supply*! A drop in the ocean. We're probably getting more oestrogen just from drinking our tap water!

Unless you have hormone receptive cancer, such as breast cancer, or are bleeding from the vagina or uterus without good cause, there should be no barrier to being offered a *repeated* prescription of local oestrogen. Even if you do suffer from the conditions mentioned, it isn't an immediate rule-out but rather a place to start your discussions. I've heard of many women who have survived breast cancer and who are left with horrific vaginal atrophy as a result of chemotherapy and have decided to use local oestrogen or take HRT irrespective of the potential consequences. For them, *quality* of life is important. And in fact, experts now agree that local oestrogen is safe to use by women who have had breast cancer in the past.

If you're already on HRT and you're being refused local oestrogen because 'you can't double up on hormone replacements', you can tell your doctor it's utter hogwash. Ask them to direct you to the medical research that informed them of that decision and then look into it yourself to make sure they aren't following the *incorrect* findings of a disastrous 2002 report that we'll turn to in Chapter 5. The sheer number of women I speak to who have been refused this treatment for no medically valid reason is concerning. Which brings me on to my second worry.

I think this patch-it-up method of giving women very short treatment or of refusing it entirely says a lot about the way the condition is generally regarded: as something that is a fleeting inconvenience that a little cream can't fix. I wish some of the medical profession would join one of my support groups, or sit down and properly talk to a woman with

VA to understand just how life-changing it is. Similarly, I wish all women suffering with VA would speak openly about it so that their doctors have some chance of gaining an insight. We can't expect things to improve if we aren't willing to engage with the process.

And perhaps just as worrying is how few women, if they are lucky enough to be prescribed local oestrogen, are being given physical examinations even after months of using the medication and seeing no improvement. It's wonderful that their doctors have suddenly developed x-ray eyes but I don't think it would hurt to pop their head down there just to check everything is OK. How do they know that there's nothing more serious going on? Of course, if your medical history is very clear and straightforward, your doctor might not need to physically examine you on your first visit, but if your symptoms don't improve, you should question why they aren't having a look.

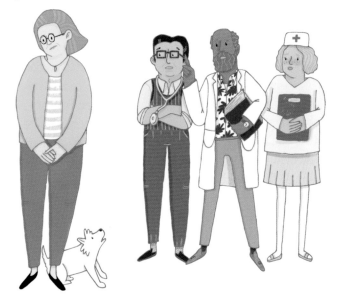

And though of course a medical professional is (hopefully) much more knowledgeable than you are *medically*, you probably also know more about your body than you think you do. If something doesn't look right, feel right or smell right, it probably isn't right, and no amount of doctor reassurance should automatically override your intuition.

Luckily for me, I didn't have this problem; my doctor has always been very patient, supportive and empathic with my condition, giving me the time and space to really discuss my options. But that doesn't go to say that every person I've seen has been like that. Far from it. I've spent lots of money on my credit card seeing some very highly regarded medical professionals, only to be met with eye-rolls, heavy sighs and dismissive remarks – being told even to 'use it or lose it' when describing the absolute agony of living with VA and trying to have sex. In fact, even as I'm writing this, a woman has just posted online the advice her doctor has given her about dealing with sex and VA: "*drink a bottle of wine to relax and see a counsellor.*" For me, this advice is disgusting and I think even deserves reporting to the General Medical Council. How *dare* someone give such negligent advice to a woman who is so clearly in both physical and emotional pain? It makes my blood boil.

So whilst I have always had an excellent GP, *my problem* was that my vulva just wasn't cooperating whenever I went to see her. Every time I went for an appointment to discuss the steady decline of my VA, my vulva looked so plump and springy you could practically trampoline off it. It was obviously a bit tricky therefore for my doctor to really see what I was complaining about. I knew, through my daily self-examination, that some days my vulva was so red, it looked like a tomato. And that other days, it would be white and almost thick. Others, it was split and bleeding, with micro cuts all over the vestibule and perineum. She never saw any of these and, well, it started to irritate me.

And so that's when I established the Vaparrazi: a daily photographer (aka my husband: hired by force) to document the many faces of my angry vulva.

Every morning and night, either I or my husband would take a picture of my genitalia on my phone, to create a more accurate picture of what I was having to deal with, the idea being that I'd be able to take them later to the doctor as 'evidence'. If you ever want to really test the love and commitment of your relationship, I think sending your partner down the vulval-mines with nothing but a phone torch-light and a message of good will, will just about do the trick.

Eventually, when I went back to the doctor with no improvement of my VA, I handed her my phone so she could see how much I was suffering. Because, unlike a penis which would be so visually obvious if it had anything resembling VA, our pain is hidden away. Unless we go out of our way therefore to reveal the issue, it can sometimes feel like our problems are being overlooked. If a man went to see his GP with a red, dry and split penis, I'm not sure he would've been told to have a drink and relax before having sex.

And I mean, on the outside, I looked fine. I could wear my nice clothes, put on a smile, tell a few jokes and seem OK. If I start talking about my pain, then, it can seem a bit exaggerated or perhaps only incidental to my life. But if you saw these pictures, you would understand the pain I was going through. You would understand that I was suffering. And that the constant soreness and burning feels sometimes like I'm being stung by a hive of bees or am rubbing salt and vinegar crisps into a cracked and split lip. That the soreness is so sharp and almost high-pitched that it's sometimes all I can do to stay sane and not throw things at people. That at one point, the skin on my vulva and perineum was so delicate that if I made a sudden move on a chair, it risked splitting open – like a moth's wing caught in glue.

And so, by seeing these pictures, you'd realise that VA wasn't likely to be cured with a short spritz of cream and that perhaps something else also needed to be done to help mend the area. You'd also know that telling us just to get on with our lives, to get drunk and have sex and forget about the VA would be possibly the *worst* thing you could say and that maybe instead directing us to some more appropriate forms of treatment would be better. For example, a women's health physiotherapist, rather than the bottle.

Women's Health Physiotherapy

I had never in my life heard of a women's health physiotherapist (we'll call them WHPs) until I had a vagina that needed fixing. How exactly was it different to a normal physiotherapist? Was it just a gimmicky advertising thing that slapped 'women's' on the front, like they do with pink razors, but ultimately was no different to the regular ones?

Oh no. No, no, *no*.

Now, I'm not really religious but to me WHPs are angels in disguise. They've helped me out in so many ways – I can't imagine the state I'd be in if I hadn't been to see them. Of course, I'm still suffering – I'm not sure if anything will change that now – but from the care and attention given to me from weekly, and then monthly sessions, I've made huge improvements in my vulvovaginal health. There may be many reasons why a WHP might be good for you, not just for VA: maybe you can't have sex, maybe you're leaking a bit, maybe you're in constant discomfort. Whatever it is, heading to your WHP is a great place to start. It's the equivalent to having a vaginal MOT.

So what is it exactly that they do?

Because this is an area that a lot of women know very little about or are too embarrassed to pursue, I think it's worth taking a bit of time to detail what you might expect from such sessions so that hopefully it will encourage you to have a go yourself.

This type of physio feels a bit like the love child of a smear test and a massage, but with more having been inherited from the latter than the former. Each treatment will usually involve a gentle internal massage of the vagina walls which, whilst might not sound all that relaxing, is likely to relieve you from a lot of pain and tension. By internally releasing points of pressure and tightness, they're bringing back blood flow to the area which in turn helps to reduce pain and discomfort. They're trying to get the old machine working again by cranking it up and keeping it well oiled.

When you first meet your WHP, they'll take a full medical history and will ask you specific vulvovaginal related questions. Please be honest here, ladies. I hear of so many women who can't bring themselves to disclosing the full extent of their symptoms for fear of embarrassment. Don't be shy, tell all.

At your first appointment, you'll be asked to get undressed down to your bra and knickers and your WHP will check out your general structure from the front, back and sides of your body – basically seeing how well you've been put together. With your underwear still on, they'll ask you to lie down on the bed and will have a feel of your muscle tone on the outside of your body – especially around your tummy and bum area. This isn't a test to see how far you can suck in your stomach, let it all hang out like the gloriously doughy splodge it probably is.

So far, all good.

They'll then give you a small towel and ask you to take off your knickers, dropping open your legs like a preying mantis. With the towel still over you, in order to maintain your dignity, they'll have a gentle root around in the nooks and crannies of your vulva like a mechanic under the bonnet of a car. This allows them to get an idea of the skin quality around your vulva and gives them a good indication of what things might be like internally. Many more serious vulval skin conditions, like lichen sclerosus, can also be detected through this thorough examination and so, even though it might make you at the thought of it cringe, it's a good idea to go.

Once your WHP has perhaps spent longer around your bits than your partner has for a while, they'll put on a glove, lube up and gently guide one finger into your vagina – very softly feeling their way around the muscles of your vaginal walls to test for tone, elasticity and any areas of tension that might be causing you problems. Once inside, the WHP will ask you to do a series of very simple exercises to test your muscle tone and pelvic floor i.e is it too tense, too weak or, like Goldilocks' porridge, just right? They'll be checking to see if there's any sign of tension that needs releasing or even prolapse that needs correcting.

It wasn't until I started having physio sessions myself that I really understood the importance of the pelvic floor – I thought it was for slim, leotard clad gym-bunnies to worry about, or for women who have just had a baby and wanted to tighten back up. The thought of my pelvic floor didn't really cross my mind.

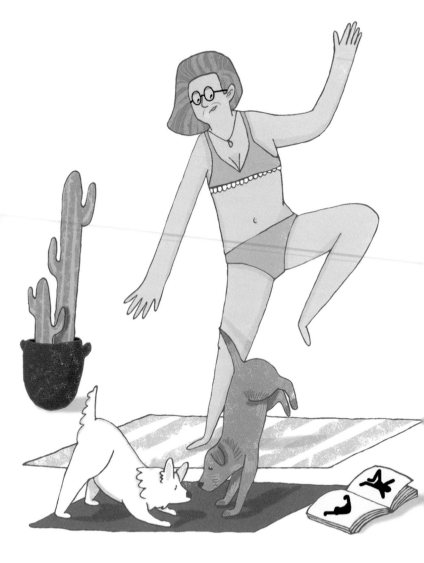

Until I was given homework.

And by homework, I mean the *physical* work I was set each week by my WHP to ensure I was tightening back up the muscles that had become too sloppy, and relaxing those that had become too tense. I think that we have become a bit too focused on the need to *tighten* our pelvic floors – many a yoga and Pilates instructor has told my daughters to squeeze, squeeze, squeeze that pelvic muscle, but I'm not sure how many people give enough focus on the *relaxing* of it. This is vitally important. If we see our pelvic muscles as a bit like a lacy bra holding up our boobs, we'll realise that if our bra is too loose, we're not supported properly and so start dropping down but that if it's too tight, we eventually start to ache and feel uncomfortable. The same goes for our pelvic muscles: they must be relaxed enough to let *all* our wee out, but tight enough to stop the valve and prevent us from leaking. Many morning routines were spent sprawled naked on the landing with my little dogs looking suspiciously at me as I tried to squat without bending my spine and raise my leg without lifting my hip. I became aware of whole parts of my body I didn't even know existed and started feeling looser in places I had long since forgotten.

You see, I had no idea that some of my symptoms could actually be improved by simple exercises. Did *you* know that the majority of women who leak a bit of pee when they're laughing or coughing can actually be cured, or at least helped, by seeing a WHP? The figures are staggering and the evidence is there if you take the time to search for it on the internet. We seem to have accepted that peeing ourselves is somehow part and parcel of being a menopausal, or even postnatal, woman. It's almost become something we *laugh* about. "Oh, I just peed myself a little, hehehe", we say, as though losing control of our bladder is somehow funny. Is it? We seem to slap on the incontinence pads as though they're an inevitability and continue as though it's all perfectly normal. This seems strange. It might *well* be the case that we need to use incontinence pads – and if we do, then we thank our lucky stars that we have something to help us, but I think it should be more routine practice to deal with the root of the problem than just try to plaster over the symptoms.

By visiting a WHP, you'll learn how to use your pelvic floor properly and will be directed to practices and/or products that might help you in your recovery of VA or other conditions. It even helped the daughter of a friend of mine who had severe endometriosis and found it very painful to have sex, so you could discuss it with your friends and family as something they might want to consider. I'd say that WHPs alone helped my VA significantly. They directed me to products I now rely on everyday and showed me how to use dilators to keep the vagina open and healthy. I'll talk about these a bit later.

What's actually really worrying is the sheer number of women I've spoken to who have been offered vaginal mesh to help with their incontinence or vaginal prolapse *before* being signposted to a WHP. Whilst this procedure aims to strengthen the weaker organs, and has been successful for many women, there are thousands of women who have had unsuccessful mesh repairs and who have suffered terribly as a result, at times even being worse off than they were *before* the surgery.

What's going on? Not only is this expensive for either the NHS or for you, but it's also potentially risky and has proven to have devastating consequences for some women who have undergone the 'small' surgery. Luckily, with campaigns like *Sling the Mesh*, such evidently barbaric procedures are starting to become a thing of the past and many fabulous doctors are now dedicating their medical practice solely to correcting some of the lasting negative impacts. Before you think about mesh surgery, I would really recommend seeing your WHP who might be able to help improve the prolapse by giving you exercises to do or perhaps even suggesting you use vaginal pessaries. Despite popular belief, these are not just for elderly ladies but have proven to be really effective for women of every age. In fact, I know of a 20 year old who has just had a baby and is finding the pessary really helpful. These pessaries come in all shapes and sizes and your WHP should be able to direct you to a suitable one. If you've had mesh and are in a bit of a state, don't lose hope but *do* get in touch with a doctor who can help you properly. Don't suffer in silence.

But what gets to me is that this trend of offering vaginal mesh or short course treatments to desperate women says a lot about where our focus is: on providing *quick fixes* rather than *long term solutions*. We see it in our treatment of new mothers, even. How is it that we can expect a woman to birth new life, rip herself open, be sewn back up, and be home on the sofa all within a few hours? If a man had his penis torn open from the tip to his bumhole, would he really be sent on his way with little else than an encouraging smile and a thumbs up for good luck? If I'd been encouraged to see a WHP after the birth of my three children, or if I'd used local oestrogen to help heal my episiotomies, I'm sure I wouldn't have been in the state I'm in.

Perhaps, because of our stoicism and willingness to just *get on with it*, we've almost made a rod for our own backs

– expecting and accepting pain as and when it comes. If we were a little more vocal and were the cheerleaders of our own lives, we might be able to change this mindset. Start by changing your mindset. Talk about your pain. Ask for help.

So, please ladies, do not consider vaginal mesh until you've thoroughly researched the pros and cons of such a procedure and *only* until you've explored every other avenue.

Try oestrogen. Visit your WHP. Perhaps, even, consider laser treatment.

Vaginal Laser Treatment

The third time I had my vagina lasered, I did a fanny fart in the doctor's face.

It was so loud and so full of gumption that we both froze for several seconds, figuring out whether we should be professional and pretend it never happened or piss ourselves laughing. We went for the latter and exploded in hysterics. I was mortified.

It's a strange thing to consider lasering your vagina, and even stranger actually getting it done. From my research online and from hearing women discussing it on different forums, I'd been aware of vaginal laser treatment for several years before I actually started thinking seriously about it. It seemed like a last-chance saloon and looked incredibly expensive, with procedures averaging at around £1500, so for a long time it didn't really feel like a legitimate option. As I'd given up my job due to VA, I simply didn't have that kind of money. And anyway I was really worried that it would make my burning much worse, rather than soothe it. It went against everything that felt natural to apply something so hot to something already inflamed.

But as I started to watch other women have a go and come out the other end unscathed, and even improved, I became more and more interested and eventually when my condition became unbearable I decided to look into it more seriously.

From what I could see, the idea behind this treatment was that the laser would help to stimulate the production of collagen in the vulvovaginal area which would therefore rejuvenate the atrophied tissue and spring it back to life. By plumping it back up, the area would have more elasticity and hydration and would therefore feel less delicate and prone to tearing. It sounded a bit like basting a Sunday chicken in its own juices to prevent it from getting too dry. Every professional offering the laser treatment claimed that it wouldn't hurt and that it would be only minimally invasive: no surgery, no lasting side-effects, and no pain.

Other than the price, it sounded too good to be true. But I was desperate and so I decided to give it a go – after all, if lasers worked miracles on eyes, maybe they could would work miracles on my vagina.

Perhaps rather unusually, my daughter came along to the first few appointments, meeting me in London to BBQ my bits. I've been incredibly lucky to have had the support of a wonderful family and they've always come along to support me when they can. I'd urge you all to share your suffering so that you can get help too. We both sat listening to the risks (it might feel sore, it might not improve the atrophy) and benefits (it might improve the atrophy) before I took off my knickers and popped behind a screen where the doctor was waiting with a small machine and what looked like a pair of curling tongs attached to it.

Because I'd gotten myself into a bit of state about the possibilities of it making my atrophy *worse*, I began to cry and started to panic. I couldn't imagine being able to cope with any more pain and so the fact that there was a *risk* it could intensify before it got better really scared me. If there was one image that could sum up those first horrific years of atrophy it would be that: of me lying on a bed with no knickers on, crying, desperate to try anything to make the pain stop. But after a lot of patience and kind words, the doctor reassured me that it was a low-risk procedure and that many women didn't even feel the effects of the laser. With a deep breath, I lay back down and opened my legs, feeling very vulnerable indeed.

Holding the laser 'wand', the doctor inserted it gently into my vagina. Due to the nature of the procedure, the doctor warned me that she couldn't use lubrication to help ease it in, so there was a bit of discomfort at first, but as it was only about as thick as a thumb, it wasn't too bad.

Once inside, the doctor moves the wand slowly around – making sure it's reaching the furthermost depths of your vagina – zapping everything in its way. Don't worry about it going up too far – it has a cap on the top to prevent it from reaching your cervix. My VA was so bad that the doctor found it difficult to turn the wand smoothly around, finding there was quite a lot of resistance from the lack of lubrication inside. Luckily for me, I didn't feel any pain at all from this internal lasering and only felt a very slight vibration coming from the wand itself. After about 60 seconds it was done! So fast!

The doctor did explain that for the first treatment the laser settings would be turned to low, so that your body and skin can get used to it and that therefore the next two visits

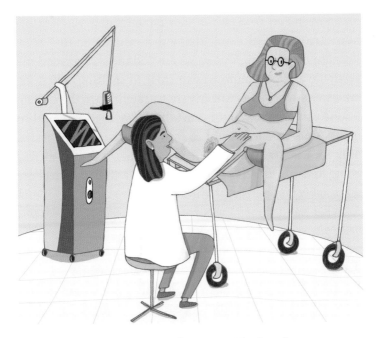

might feel more intense, but considering how nervous I was and how much I had worked myself up, I was pleasantly surprised.

But then she started on my vulva.

After again changing the cap on the wand to suit the outer area, the doctor got to work zapping everything she could between my legs. The fragility and thinning of my vulva skin was one of the main reasons I decided to get laser treatment and so I knew that was likely to cause me the most pain. In fact, because my episiotomy scars had atrophied and tightened so much, it was agonising to walk or do anything at all really, including sitting or lying down. It felt like my labia was tissue paper, ready to rip at any moment.

Although the internal lasering was pain free, the external was a slightly different story. If you've ever burnt your skin on an oven tray or a pair of hair straighteners you'll know how sore it can feel – well, that was how it felt on my vulva. Because my scarring was so severe and the skin around my vestibule and perineum was so close to splitting, when the laser went over it I very nearly shot straight up to the ceiling. I don't usually swear but I don't think I've ever said *Shit!* so many times in one breath! Even though the zapping lasted only for one minute, once it had finished I felt like I was going to throw up, the pain was intense and I could feel my scars, labia and perineum throbbing.

What had I done? I was panicking – *please don't let this be it, please don't let this be it*.

But after about 20 minutes, as if by magic, the pain from the laser almost miraculously stopped and the more general soreness I'd been living with for all those years before returned. It felt like welcoming back an old friend. I guess in some ways I was a bit disappointed that there wasn't an immediate cure, even though I knew *logically* that it wasn't the way the procedure worked, there was a part of me that was hoping for that *ta-dah* moment when the pain would be suddenly and completely lifted from me. But the doctor was very good at explaining the process and of reassuring me that it would take time for the tissue to regenerate.

After the procedure, they tell you to take it easy for a few days but unluckily for me I had to run for my train (worrying that my vagina was going to fall out as I ran) and then once on it, stand all the way home – wishing dearly that there was a 'Burning Vagina On Board' badge to wear so I could get a seat (but then also realising that even if I got it I wouldn't be able to sit down anyway). As soon as I got back, I went straight to my bedroom and took out my magnified mirror to see the state of my vulva post-lasering.

Wow. What a sight.

Red raw, covered in what looked like minuscule pin-pricks, my vulva resembled what I'd imagine two slugs to look like after being out in the sun all day and then run over. It wasn't a pretty sight, but then it hadn't been for a long time, so what could I expect?

For the next three days I pottered around my street knickerless, walking like John Wayne and took great delight in telling my neighbours I'd had my vagina lasered when they asked me what was wrong. If you have concerned neighbours and want the conversation to end smartish, I'd recommend having the treatment just for that!

On day four, the soreness had nearly died down and I felt pleased with having survived the laser wand. Although I wouldn't say I noticed a massive improvement in the next few weeks, my skin no longer felt like it was going to rip whenever I walked or sat and so for that alone I was grateful.

In order for the treatment to work properly, I knew I had to go back between two to four more times so that it would allow the skin to stimulate the collagen that it so desperately needed. And so, six weeks later I trotted back to London and BBQ'd my vagina once more. The second and third times were much less painful and after each one I started to really notice the improvement in skin quality and elasticity. Even though I was still sore from the atrophy, I no longer felt fragile or delicate or that I was at risk of suddenly splitting open. For most people, three laser treatments is enough to maximise the benefits but because my episiotomy scars were so deep and long, I ended up having five – the last two were focused just on my outer skin.

I'd say that the laser treatment, though expensive, did improve my symptoms by quite a lot. I guess it felt like the difference between wearing a pair of shoes that gave you blisters and then putting on trainers; though ultimately we would like slippers, they're comfy enough.

When I went back to my WHP she said that if she hadn't known the vagina was mine, she would've thought it belonged to a woman in her mid-twenties; the plumpness and skin quality was so improved she could hardly believe it was the same one. Though perhaps the skin *looks* better than it feels, I'm so glad I had it done and wish I'd had the courage and the insight to do it earlier.

If you're considering vaginal laser treatment but are worried about it, based on my own experiences I'd recommend it. Of course, this procedure will not be suitable or appropriate for everyone and you should always do your own research before you consider any type of treatment but in my case, I was glad I had it done. It didn't *cure* me but it did help. Definitely make sure you're visiting a professional, though, who really knows what they're doing.

Of the women I know who have also had it done, I'd say that the majority have noticed either a slight or a big improvement in their vulvovaginal health and that only a small number have had no improvement. I also know this procedure is working especially well for women with lichen sclerosus or for those who have finished chemotherapy, so I think it should definitely be something you consider or talk to your doctor or specialist about. It *is* expensive but there are so many 0% credit cards out there at the moment that allow you to borrow for many months that the monthly payback isn't too bad. Hopefully one day this treatment will be fully quality assured and more readily available to us.

In fact, a vaginal laser treatment called *Mona Lisa Touch* is currently being used as a trial in the NHS, so there's hope!

And so, once a year for the rest of my life, I'll be trotting back to London to laser my vagina, hoping with all my heart that when my daughter's are my age access to this treatment will have greatly improved.

CHAPTER 5

HRT and Local Oestrogen

This chapter might do well to begin with the conclusion: I am not pro-HRT, I am pro-choice. Like the drug itself, I am sure the words within this chapter are likely to divide opinion. But that's OK because discussion is healthy, and so is disagreement. So long as we're educating ourselves beyond the headlines, debate can only make things better.

~

My life before and after HRT

Today, I feel like myself. Or at least *more* like myself. This is pretty significant because seven years ago I couldn't imagine ever feeling like myself again. I've just come back from taking Bertie and Bonnie for a walk and was able to wear knickers and trousers all the way round. This is a small miracle. Even though I'm now sitting on a heat pad with my legs spread trying to soothe the dull ache from my vulva, the very fact that I *sat* in a car and wore *knickers* and *trousers* and *walked*, all in one morning I think deserves a bit of a celebration. If I were a drinker, I might even pour myself a glass and raise a toast to my vagina.

You see, the thing is, unless you've experienced vaginal atrophy yourself and understand just how debilitating it can be, it's difficult to really get across how it feels to live with it every day.

I guess it would be like wearing a pair of new leather shoes, with no socks, and being made to run a marathon. Imagine that at some point along the way, a small stone finds its way down the back of them and starts rubbing away at your heel. At the start, it's just annoying – you make vague attempts to brush the grit from your foot but ultimately you're OK. But after a while, when you still haven't managed to get it out and its dug and dug and dug away at the skin, it becomes a *significant* problem and it's suddenly all you can think about. It's taken over your mind as well as your body. You're not who you used to be because you can't seem to focus on anything else.

I'm sure you can imagine how this would feel and how much you would want to stop running and remove them. But the thing is, you can't. The most you can do is walk slowly, rest now and then and accept that your feet will continue to be blistered and throbbing in pain. You might find some nice walkers along the way who stop to see if you're OK or walk along slowly next to you, but for the most part, they see you as a bit of an annoyance and wonder why you're making such a fuss. After all, their feet are completely fine.

Living with vaginal atrophy is like trying to finish a race with blistered feet: raw, swollen, stinging. Even though you know you have to keep going, and that your feet are only a small part of your body and so shouldn't really be causing you this much hassle, it's all you can do to stay upright. The thought of you being able to simply forget about the pain is almost laughable. Or at least it would be if you still had a sense of humour.

Because the problem with chronic pain is that after a while things stop being funny. Even your positivity, which you've tried so hard to maintain, starts to dwindle and irritates you. In fact, *everything* irritates you. The fact that you're always irritated irritates you. When you've tried everything, and nothing seems to work, all you want to do is wallow in the rubbish reality of your rubbish situation and stay there. Life is a bitch and therefore you are too.

During the darkest days of my vaginal atrophy, I really couldn't see the wood for the trees. I felt like I had literally tried everything to soothe the pain: homeopathy, moisturisers, yoga, meditation, hypnotherapy. I found nothing that helped. The only pleasure in my day came from the thought of bedtime, when I knew there might be a few stolen moments when my pain would cease.

For a while, I had heard from others about this drug called HRT and how it had helped them. But for years, this was just background noise, I knew it was there but ultimately it had nothing to say. *HRT is dangerous*, I thought. *Everyone knows that.* Why on earth would I take a drug that could give me breast cancer? Or poison my body with chemicals? Or increase my chance of stroke or heart attack? I was desperate, not deranged (although, actually, at that point, that's perhaps debatable)!

But once all your options have disappeared, you find that your morals start to disappear too.

And that's how I came to HRT: desperate.

HRT, they said, could help with menopausal symptoms, including hot flushes, mood swings, night sweats and vaginal atrophy. *Including* vaginal atrophy? Interesting. Although I still didn't like the thought of being on a drug for the rest of my life, I knew I couldn't go on as I was either.

And so, with unwashed hair, tear-stained cheeks and desperately low morale, I dragged myself to the GP and asked about my options. I felt like I had sold out or that I was asking for Class A Drugs. I never thought I'd be the type of person to give in so easily.

Only 10 minutes later, and I came out holding a prescription for HRT. One month later, my pubes started coming back. Two months later, my vulva started plumping back up. Three months later, *I* started coming back.

For me, the benefits were pretty significant. For months, my shins, eyes and ears had been so unbearably itchy that most nights I'd be manically scratching them until they bled – with HRT that all stopped. In numerous places around my body, including my nose and perineum, I had extremely sore micro-cuts which seemed never to heal and always caused me discomfort – with HRT they went away. Every night I'd get up between 3-4 times to go for a wee and had a constant pain in my bladder area – with HRT these nightly toilet trips reduced to only one and my bladder felt much calmer. My hay fever which developed very late in life and which caused me no end of suffering in the summer, disappeared. My pubic and armpit hair grew back, becoming almost so thick I needed to plait it or use a lawn mower to trim it down. The skin around my clitoral hood had for many months become so atrophied and shrivelled that it had pulled right back, permanently exposing the sensitive clitoris underneath and making it unbearable to wear knickers – with HRT it plumped back up and protected the area as it should. My anal fissures, which had bled almost every day since the birth of my first child over 30 years ago, had reduced so much in size that I could go to the toilet normally. My joints felt less achy. I slept better. I felt less blue. I still wouldn't associate myself with absolute happiness but I would no longer associate myself with suicide either. My depression became manageable and allowed me to seek help from professionals.

It is clear then, that for me, HRT was a bit of a hero. But that isn't to say I came to use it easily or that I wasn't scared of the impact it could have on my body. Of course I was and in many ways I still am, but what I know is that my life wouldn't in any way be enjoyable if I'd continued without its help.

I spent *years* of my perimenopause absolutely adamant that I wouldn't touch HRT with a barge pole. The headlines were so clear: HRT will shorten your life. One way or another, HRT would find a way to kill you, whether that be through cancer, stroke or heart attack. It wasn't *if* it damaged you, it was *how*. I simply wasn't prepared to take the risk.

But it wasn't until I started doing my own research on the medication that I started to actually understand it a bit more and to appreciate how and why it was such a political and medical hot potato.

Whether you're interested in taking HRT or not, I think it's really important to have an idea about where our societal perception of it actually came from. Everything I discuss below has been referenced at the back of the book, please do take the time to do your own research.

What is HRT?

HRT stands for hormone replacement therapy. This is because it *replaces* hormones lost as a result of menopause. The key word here is *replacement*, a concept often overlooked. If something is replaced, it simply means it is being substituted by something of the same, or very similar, kind. Usually this is because the thing being replaced is very important, otherwise we'd just forget about it and not bother.

Take Type 1 diabetes for example. When someone doesn't produce enough or any insulin naturally in their body, they're given it artificially because there's an understanding that insulin is a hormone needed in order for the body to be healthy.

The same goes for menopause.

When we reach menopausal age, our biological purpose of growing, birthing and feeding babies ceases and with it goes the hormones necessary to aid that reproduction. But, of course, those hormones were not only essential in the creation and maintenance of *new* life, they were also vitally important in the maintenance of *your* life.

Let's take oestrogen.

Now, oestrogen is the hormone that gives us boobs, pubes and those much loved child bearing hips when we're going through puberty; it also helps our bodies to regulate periods. If we don't get pregnant, our oestrogen levels plummet and we bleed. If we do get pregnant, oestrogen hooks up with progesterone to prevent us from ovulating during the pregnancy and helps our breasts produce milk to feed the little sprog when we eventually squeeze it out.

Crucially, however, oestrogen is also vital in the building and maintaining of other areas of our body, not least our bones. Working together with calcium, vitamin D and other hormones, oestrogen ensures our skeleton is stable and our bones are healthy. When we reach menopause, due to the lack of these bone-building hormones, our bodies start to break down more bone matter than we produce, leaving us more susceptible to osteoporosis. We become a bit like a well-played game of Jenga: one wrong move and we're a jumbled mess on the floor.

As well as bones and bleeds, oestrogen also helps to keep the rest of our bodies fit and healthy: from the maintenance of our skin and hair to the proper functioning of our pelvic muscles and brain cells, affecting not just the mechanics but also the mood of the body and mind. In short, chronically low oestrogen levels can make us feel pretty grotty, both physically and emotionally.

The same goes for testosterone.

It might surprise you to learn that testosterone is actually a pretty big deal in women's bodies and that, in fact, without testosterone our bodies wouldn't be able to produce oestrogen. Low testosterone levels in a woman's body have not only been linked with bone and muscle loss, potential cardiovascular and cognitive problems but also issues with the vagina, including atrophy and loss of libido. Unfortunately for me, I can't seem to take testosterone without having undesired side effects, but for others it can make you feel more energised and less depressed.

It's no wonder then that without some of these essential hormones, our bodies start choking and find it difficult to function, and so someone thought it a good idea to come up with something to help fix the mess.

Enter HRT stage left. Like fertiliser to a dying plant, it was realised that if we wanted to stay healthy and strong we might need to give ourselves the right nutrients to do so. Otherwise, we might just start wilting.

HRT, then, simply acts as a *replacement* to these hormones lost through menopause, the very hormones that we've just seen as being integral to the proper functioning of our bodies. The job of HRT isn't to fill our bodies with hormones it's not used to; on the contrary, it aims to refuel our bodies with the hormones it's not used to being *without*. From the women I've spoken to on my forum, I think this is where a lot of the misconception lies: in the idea that our bodies are *natural* as they are, and that by using HRT, we're adding something *unnatural* to them.

Now, remember ladies, in the grand scheme of things, it's been only until relatively recently that we women have actually *survived* for so long in life. Even if we look at the global rising trend of life expectancy in women, we can see that already we're living 10-15 years longer than our grandparents and it looks like this figure will continue to rise. But of course, though we may be *living* longer, that's in no way a clear indication of how *healthy* we are when we reach these 'gained' years. With every 80 or 90 year old woman who's survived an extra 10 years to that of her grandmother, there's an 80 or 90 year old vagina sitting along with her, most likely suffering from severe atrophy and most probably very uncomfortable. I'm not sure, therefore, what is natural or unnatural at this stage but if we're expecting our bodies to keep us ticking over for longer than they'd signed up for, it seems likely that they might need a little helping hand to prevent them from giving up the ghost entirely.

Media vs medicine

But for some, being able to have an open and unbiased dialogue about HRT with their GP seems to be almost impossible. This drug appears to be such a political hot-potato that for some it's turning any possibility of getting a prescription into mash.

And yet, as far as I can see, medication is dished out rather willingly for other age-related symptoms: osteoporosis, Alzheimer's, Parkinson's, heart attacks, arthritis. For these conditions, we seem quite happy to offer something to help.

And rightly so. No one should be made to live in pain or discomfort if there's no need to.

In fact, if we go one stage further and start looking at our willingness to dish out medication for *comfort* or *quality of experience* or *enjoyment* you'll see that we're actually pretty happy to do that too. I mean, let's look at Viagra.

This little blue pill has become something of a star in its own right, jokingly referred to amongst friends, in films and even advertised freely in magazines and newspapers. Simply type in *Viagra* into Google and you'll have no problem at all getting your hands on it. In fact, it's so easy to get hold of, it seems to be almost encouraged. We accept that sex is important and that without it, it might cause some physical or emotional strain on a person's wellbeing. We're happy therefore to help a broken penis. But a vagina? Hmm. We're not so sure. Perhaps my view is overly simplistic but it seems troubling that medication to treat erectile dysfunction can be so easily obtained without a prescription, but that HRT requires hoops, hurdles and rainbows to jump over before it's granted. Both relate to a person's ability to enjoy a full and healthy life (not just in respect of sex) and have control over their bodies. Both are for adults who presumably know the consequences of taking such medication.

Both are there to correct something that isn't working properly. Why are we happy to give men a pill to help their penis without first investigating the reasons *behind* the dysfunction? Perhaps the argument is that Viagra is taken as a one off and has a limited physiological effect on the body, but I know of many women whose husbands take it as a regular and as there's no barrier to buying it freely, then it's likely that many others will be too.

It can sometimes feel, then, that for menopause there are too many *barriers* to medication and that these barriers are based more on politics than medicine.

Talk to only a small handful of women of menopausal age about HRT, and I can almost guarantee you'll be met with some very emotional and confused responses; most women are afraid of the drug but aren't sure exactly why, adamant they won't touch it and even wary of those who do. I think this fear is fed by the horror stories greedily gobbled up by the media and spat out to sell newspapers, giving far too much stage time to potential side effects and not enough time to present the *facts* in a non-biased way. Where are the stories of the women whose lives have improved since taking the drug? Where's the neutral reporting of the benefits as well as the potential consequences? We're not stupid – we know that *all* drugs have side effects, but it does seem peculiar that this is a case where the benefits are in some instances completely overlooked by the very women who should be taking it.

So where did this fear of hormone replacement therapy come from? To answer this, we must first briefly cast our minds back to the swinging sixties.

Clinical trials

Now, in the mid-60s, when HRT was first introduced in the UK, it enjoyed a very welcoming reception; menopausal women were finally able to revel in the joys of hormone balance and a higher quality of life. Along with its sister, the contraceptive pill, women were suddenly given the tools to control their bodies, minds and subsequently their lives, allowing them to enjoy a life with more freedom, independence and enjoyment. With the contraceptive pill still being one of the most readily available and politically neutral drugs, our acceptance of *some* hormone treatments has continued even today. For others it's a very different story.

Four decades later, and the HRT vibes start to sour. Without getting too bogged down in the details, this sudden change came about as a result of a 2002 clinical trial that found an increased risk of breast cancer in *some* women if taken over a long period of time. This headline-snappy anecdote trail-blazed its way through the media like a fox in a hen-barn: ruffling feathers and causing chaos and destruction in its wake. Reporters up and down the country took to their perch and crowed endlessly about the harms of HRT and for many, many years not much was said about its benefits. Women stopped taking it. Doctors stopped prescribing it. For someone like me who has benefited so much from HRT, this kind of scaremongering could have come between me and my health and happiness.

The problem with this clinical trial was that the findings were misleading. Frankly, as far as I can see, the whole investigation seemed a bit dodgy. Although the results indicated a small increased risk of diseases such as breast cancer, heart disease, blood clots and stroke in some women in this study, what the media failed to publicise were the details of the women actually taking part in the trial. These details were crucial.

Whilst I'd absolutely advise you to read the full report to gain your own understanding (see back of book for details), *some* of the main issues with the study have been listed below. Remember, it's this flawed report that instigated the dawn of the HRT controversy:

- The participants in the trial were women from the US, not the UK. These women were much older than the women on HRT in the UK (average age in this study was 64) and so were already at a higher risk of breast cancer, heart disease and stroke. This is because the risk of these diseases *naturally* increases with age. It was incorrect to attribute this risk solely to HRT.

- Most of the women in the trial were largely overweight. As is widely recognised now, being overweight brings an increased risk of heart disease and some cancers. This includes breast cancer. The reported increased risk of breast cancer therefore couldn't be attributed to HRT any more than the factor of being overweight.

- The trial wasn't randomised. The women who took part were self-selecting and self-reporting and many of them dropped out before the trial had concluded. The reporting therefore, wasn't transparent and didn't give the whole picture of the trial.

The damage, however, was done.

By 2003, everyone was confused. Doctors began to advise their patients to come off HRT, hormone-reliant women started suddenly going cold-turkey and the media continued to reel out propaganda that sold newspapers but didn't serve the people. As a result of this scaremongering, the amount of women taking HRT fell by more than half and left nearly 1 million women in the UK alone suffering with their symptoms in silence and without medical help. To counteract this unnecessary and potentially dangerous decline, a subsequent report was published which analysed in detail the findings of the earlier trials. Not only did they find the initially published results were overestimated and misleading, but they also found a whole heap of *benefits* that had been completely overlooked – such as the ones I experienced myself and listed above. The results also showed that younger women who took HRT in this study had a lower risk of heart disease and osteoporosis.

It's absolutely infuriating then, that so many women had to go through years of suffering without the drug they needed because of some lazy research and reporting. If the media had been a bit less biased in their headlines, or if we and the medical profession had taken the initiative to dig a bit deeper into these findings, perhaps the controversy surrounding HRT wouldn't be so embedded.

But unfortunately the ramifications of this 2002 report have been widespread, and even today women are finding it difficult getting a prescription based on this history of misinformation. If you take the time to do your own research, however, you'll find that the results from more reliable studies have since shown that taking oestrogen as a patch or gel (which is body identical) has no risk of clots and that the body identical micronised progesterone capsule has less risk of breast cancer compared to older types of HRT. When you hear the term 'body-identical' oestrogen, it basically means that the oestrogen you're given to help with your menopause symptoms has the same *molecular* structure as the oestrogen produced (and decreased) naturally in your body. In fact, body identical HRT is available on the NHS – you just have to find a doctor who understands it…

Medicine vs morality

Every day, women are coming into my online groups, desperate: they've been refused HRT multiple times by their doctors and are no longer sure what to do with their vaginal atrophy or indeed their other symptoms of menopause. They've tried everything else already. When I ask why their GP refused this medication, 9 times out of 10 the answer will be 'because they don't agree with it' or their 'a bit anti-HRT'.

There is something very wrong with that.

When did we require a doctor's *moral* approval to take a legal drug our body perhaps needs? Why does the prescription of HRT seem to be based on a doctor lottery rather than medical science?

Of course I understand the reservations of taking a drug that you might need to be on for the rest of your life. We all do. Yes, we understand that it has side effects. Like all drugs. But what I don't understand is how and why this drug has been singled out above all others and has amassed so much fear and hostility. As a society we seem pretty happy pumping our youngsters with synthetic hormones in the form of contraceptive pills but when it comes to substituting lost hormones with natural replacements later on in life we seem up in arms.

What is *really* going on here? Because I don't believe it's based purely on science.

Ladies, if you're refused HRT and think you might benefit from it, you *must* ask why; whatever the reason, go home and do your own research. It could well be that you actually shouldn't take HRT, though there are actually fewer reasons for this than you might think, but you need to make sure you understand the reason for its refusal and feel happy that the explanation is based on *science* rather than *emotion*. If your GP refuses HRT and you're not happy with the reason given, please don't cower in the corner and take no further action. Ask the doctor for the guidelines they're basing their refusal on. Do your own research. Talk to the

Practice Manager. There is so much literature out there supporting HRT that an automatic 'no' from your GP simply won't do. I've directed you to some of this literature at the back of the book. Educate yourselves. Be vocal.

But none of this is to say that I am actually pro-HRT. I am not.

As I said at the beginning of this chapter, I am pro-choice.

When I went to see my doctor, she really listened to my fears and concerns and took the time to dispel many of the media myths and gave me a very unbiased and practical understanding of the medication. I was told the benefits it was likely to give and the side effects it might cause. She allowed me to make up my own mind and directed me to numerous places where I could read more about it.

Yet even with this choice, I was scared. Although I couldn't exactly attribute my fear to anything in particular, I guess I'd absorbed the general unease around HRT: thinking it was for horses, not humans; worried that breast cancer was an almost guaranteed consequence; feeling that I was in some way being a bit pathetic.

But the reality was that my life had lost its appeal. In my darkest moments, when I couldn't bear the pain of the atrophy and the mental torments any more, I wondered what exactly the point of my life was. I had given up my job, I could only walk and stand for a few minutes before the pain of my burning vagina became too great and I didn't want to talk to my husband or family. Vaginal atrophy took me to the very limits of my mind and body.

And so I went on HRT.

Within one month, from applying the body-identical HRT gel to my thigh and from inserting local oestrogen into my vagina, I started to feel more human. My pubes, having recently shredded their last grey stragglers, were now sprouting back and my vulva, having been so dry and painfully delicate for the last three years, had suddenly plumped up so much I reckon it could have flown away had it been left untethered. The dark, dark cloud of depression was ever so gradually starting to disperse and the unbearable pain between my legs was becoming more manageable.

I think the important thing in taking HRT is that the decision is your own. Do your research, ask women about their own experiences, go to a few different doctors. Whatever you do, don't be paralysed by the propaganda or fear that seeps its way into our society. Many women I've spoken to will not even go to their doctors to discuss the options of HRT because they've been brought up knowing only the risks, rather than the benefits, of taking the drug. If we only ever read the *warning* section of our prescription leaflets, we'd probably have croaked it a long time ago.

I'm aware of the possible side effects of taking this drug and whilst I wish on every star that I don't get them, I'm also pragmatic. For me, life couldn't have continued anyway so I am grateful for any quality of life I'm given. The pain is still very much there and so is the depression, but I feel I've been given a small amount of blue sky in an otherwise dark storm. This might not sound like much, but to me it's given me some of my life back.

I can walk again. I can wear underwear. I smile. I laugh. I cry, but not for too long. I can take my dogs across the fields. I can visit my daughters. I can cuddle my granddaughter on my lap. And so for me, that's worth it.

CHAPTER 6

Physical and Mental Wellbeing

But as well as the WHP, laser treatment, oestrogen and HRT, after seven years of suffering from VA, I've now come to realise the importance of maintaining a healthy physical and mental wellbeing practice. Physically, unless I eat well, gently exercise daily and stick to my strict vulvovaginal routine, I'm likely to be in much more pain than I might otherwise be. Mentally, by speaking openly about my condition to my friends, family and counsellor I've been able to avoid the very, very dark days I had at the beginning of my journey and have started to even have some moments of real joy. And though I know social media is getting a lot of wrap at the moment because of its addictiveness or its apparent decimation of real-life friendships, without the support of all the incredibly strong and brave women on my online forums I'm not sure how I would have weathered the storm or where I may have washed up.

If I want to have *any* resemblance of normality in my life, I have to use full HRT and local oestrogen, visit my WHP every three months, have my vagina lasered yearly and stick strictly to my daily routines. In case it's any help at all, I've detailed below the intricacies of these routines. Pick and choose what speaks to you and feel free to skip this section entirely if you've already got yours sorted.

Physical wellbeing: my vulvovaginal daily routine

As one who never wore makeup or even gave two thoughts about moisturisers, I think it's safe to say I've caught up on missed time; but rather than applying red lippy to feel glamorous, I'm applying cream to soothe my red lips! Life has a funny way of balancing itself doesn't it?

As you may have noticed, just like when you stop moisturising your dry face or hands, the ageing skin on your vulva also becomes dry and is in need of moisture. Think back to that rather sad looking house plant whose withering leaves are in desperate need of some TLC. We basically need to take a watering can to our famished shrub and use a bit of fertilizer to replenish lost nutrients.

But beware.

What you put onto your vulva and into your vagina is *very*, *very* important. As a rule, no product should go into your vagina unless you've had your doctor's OK. Before we start looking at the things we *could* use to help with our atrophy, let's eliminate the things we mustn't:

- **Don't douche**. This is rule 101 of vaginal maintenance. By forcing water into your vagina you're not only putting yourself at risk of infection, you're also getting rid of all the good bacteria your vagina has been so busy making. I'm not sure how douching became so popular and *normal* in our society, but it feels to me like another bit of pressure for women to be all nicely packaged, floral scented and hair-removed Barbie dolls. Apparently we don't fart and we don't poo. '*Vaginas should smell like roses*': what utter nonsense. Vaginas should be healthy. If your partner is that concerned about your vagina smelling nice, tell them to have sex with a rose-bush.

- **Don't use scented products**. The chemicals that are used to create a nice smelling body wash or moisturiser are not good for our skin, let alone our sensitive genitals. It is very important we don't disrupt the natural pH of our vaginas by smothering it in artificial chemicals, in the same way we wouldn't pour petrol into our rivers. We need to look after our ecosystems. If you think you need to cover up an unpleasant smell coming from your vagina, it's probably better that you visit your doctor rather than try to self-treat. It could be that you have an infection such as *bacterial vaginosis* that needs to be treated with antibiotics. Just think, if you had sun burn, you wouldn't spray perfume on it just so it could smell nice. The same goes for our vaginas and vulvas.

I was dismayed the other night when I saw a TV advert selling a well-known feminine cream for menopausal women, professing to be the cure for a whole myriad of vaginal and vulva problems. As great as a 'one-cream-fixes-all' treatment would be, if it sounds too good to be true, it probably is. Just because a product professes to cure you and has a nice picture of a happy-looking woman who has probably never suffered from vaginal pain ever in her life, doesn't mean it will. Especially when we look at the ingredients contained within it. We need to think really carefully about the products we're putting into and onto our bodies and should be aiming to use only the most natural moisturisers and lotions we can find. As a rule, other than prescription based treatments, the fewer the ingredients the product has, and the closer it is to Mother Nature, the better. I've included a list of the products I use at the back of the book.

As I'm sure your bank account has realised by now, menopause is *big* business. But despite how isolating and lonely vaginal atrophy can make you feel, if you just look at the sheer number of products lining our shelves and internet pages to treat such a problem, we should see that this condition is more widespread than you might think.

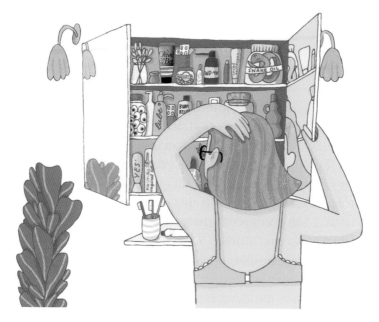

I feel pretty confident in saying that I've tried and tested most products claiming to help vaginal atrophy: some doing nothing, some helping a bit, some making it worse. My credit card has haemorrhaged money to meet the demands of my angry vagina and sadly many gels, moisturisers, and ointments have gone straight in the bin after the first application. I sometimes wish we could all just buy one product and play pass-the-parcel with them until we find one that we like, to save ourselves oodles of cash. If you have friends or a group who you think might be willing to do this, I'd suggest buying little tester pots and divvying up small amounts until you find one that works for you, otherwise be prepared to part with some coins.

My morning routine

Having slept naked all night to air the area and let the smouldering embers of the fire ease off a little[1], I usually wake up and have a shower with only water – avoiding all products that might upset the pH balance of my vulva and vagina. In my experience, even those products claiming to be pH neutral are sometimes problematic, especially if they touch an already delicate, but perhaps even inflamed, area. When I wash my hair, rather than lean my head backwards into the shower water, I'll turn around and face it with my hair falling over my face like the grim-reaper and my bum pushed right back like I'm trying to sit down. This way, I can best avoid any suds getting lodged in my nooks and crannies and I'd advise you all to do the same if you have atrophy and are very skin-sensitive. I've now even changed my shampoo and conditioner to more natural ones so that it doesn't cause me pain when it slides down my hair and onto my body.

So, I'm out the shower and like a wet dog, I shake off most of the water, patting any part of my body that's delicate or sore. It's important to be really gentle with yourself and not hurry as a rub too fast has left some of the ladies in my

---

1   I literally sleep with my butt hanging out the bed like a bungalow built too close to the cliff-edge.

support group with a tear to the skin. Looking back to when I was 40 and could dry myself so carefree with a rough towel makes me almost wince – I simply can't imagine doing that now.

Before I get dressed, I allocate around five minutes solely to my vulva. In the beginning, when I first realised I had vaginal atrophy, I'd lay on my bed completely lost, depressed and desperate about what to do. At least now I've got my routine down to a manageable amount of time. Ladies, if you're still trying to work yours out, hang on in there.

Legs akimbo and with a large magnifying mirror to hand, I apply one of three creams that I use on rotation (discussed at the end) into the vestibule area, around the labia, into the creases and on the perineum. Basically, where there is fire, I throw water.

As the products I use are oil based, they absorb throughout the day and form a *breathable* barrier to allow me to slide-and-glide and get on with my life as much as possible. Without using these moisturisers I'm in a *lot* of discomfort which sometimes feels like my clitoris has got straw lodged up it.

For me, it's really important I keep on top of any changes that are happening in my vulvovaginal area, so that's why I always make sure I have a look down there as I'm applying the creams and oils. I remember the first time I took a peek and being really shocked at what my vulva had become – '*where had it gone?*' I thought. My inner labia had reduced in size and plumpness by around 80% and the skin was so see-through it was almost like tissue-paper: hanging limply like a flag to surrender. It was by using oestrogen, HRT and applying the daily moisturisers that I began to see a huge improvement in the skin quality and started to experience a bit more comfort when walking and sitting.

Once I've applied the moisturisers and have let them sink in a little, I'll drag myself onto the floor so I can begin the exercises my WHP has set me – watching Bertie and Bonnie staring curiously at me.

With exercises done, vulva fully lubed and moisturisers popped into my handbag, I'm now ready to start the day. What a fuss!

My afternoon routine

Now that I've given up my job due to the pain of standing too long as a florist, I take my dogs for a walk across the fields to keep fit and stay sane. They are my walking meditation.

The problem I find with walking though is that it's both essential for my mental health and physical conditioning but absolutely awful for my vulva and vagina. Like a piece of grit wedged at the back of your heel on a long walk, it always ends up feeling blistered or swollen which forces me to lie down in the afternoon until it calms down. This is when I used to be most reliant on frozen baked beans cans or vegetable packs. I usually have to reapply my oil-based moisturiser at some point in the afternoon and in fact some of the ladies on my forum have to do it after each time they go to the toilet.

A word about going to the loo.

At the start, going for a wee was so painful that I'd have to take a bottle of water with me and pee-n-pour at the same time in an attempt to neutralise the sting. I couldn't use toilet paper and for a while tried the pure water-based wet-wipes but even they were too abrasive. Now I can use toilet paper again but it is a very gentle dab; even the thought of confidently wiping myself like we all used to when we were younger makes me squirm. Oh the unexpected joys of youth: being able to wipe yourself freely!

My evening routine

Before bedtime, it's important for me to have a quick squat over the bath with the shower head so that I can reapply cream again hygienically. I use local oestrogen in my vagina every other night – in the form of a pill at the end of a blue-stick plunger – and in between these nights I use one of the vaginal moisturisers I mention at the back of the book. If I'm getting extra sore through the day I'll use oestrogen cream on the outer areas of the perineum as and when necessary. I know that some ladies need to use both the vaginal moisturiser and oestrogen pill and cream every day, so again, work with what your body needs.

Unfortunately, despite wanting desperately to soak my aching joints and bones in a nice long bath, I'm no longer able to. In fact, I've not had a bath for over seven years. For me, the benefits simply don't outweigh the negatives: sore, itchy and dry skin, even if I just use water.

None of us should be bathing in chemicals anyway so please ladies really consider that bath-bomb or lathering bubble-bath that might be finding its way into your urethra or vagina and causing you jip. As I've already said, we wouldn't pour petrol into a mountain stream so don't do the same to yourselves.

Of course, sex is completely off the agenda but I've dedicated a whole section to that next so we won't go into it now. Before bed, I might do some more WHP homework by inserting a dilator into my vagina to try to keep the runway open and the vaginal muscles healthy. We'll look at that in the next chapter too.

And hurrah! I've survived another Burning Vagina Day. Off to sleep to start it all again tomorrow. What fun.

Mental wellbeing: staying sane from the pain

But as well as maintaining a strict *physical* routine, I've found keeping on top of my mental health has been just as important. After all, it's very hard to look after yourself properly if you're not in the right head space to do so.

Anyone who has ever experienced physical pain of any kind will know that it can leave you feeling sad and frustrated. You injure your knee and you start to go a bit insane from having to hobble everywhere. You have bad tooth ache and you begin to feel low from the pain of eating, talking and even sleeping. You break your arm and you feel disconnected from your body, no longer being able to do simple things like write, text or brush your teeth, lobbing a banana across the room in frustration when even that becomes impossible to peel. After a while, the mental strain of living with pain or discomfort starts to take its toll and we end up being a bit grumpy. Our temper is short and we long for a time when we feel well again.

But what happens if that pain doesn't go away? What happens if it gets worse? And what happens if people can't see what you're even complaining about?

The thing is, if we can physically *see* the pain of others, or if we have experienced it ourselves, we seem to find it easier to have empathy and patience with those who are suffering. We've all had headaches where we feel nauseous, or back ache where every step makes us squirm, or a deep cut that won't stop throbbing. If we see someone bump their broken leg on the corner of a table and shout out in pain and anger, we feel bad for them, totally understanding that it would really hurt. We don't for a second think that their anger or frustration from the pain *caused* the broken leg. That would be ridiculous.

And yet, for many women who have vaginal atrophy, one of the first things they're offered is antidepressants, suggesting that their physical condition is *as a result* of a negative state of mind. It follows then that if we changed our mindset, our labia would plump back up, our oestrogen levels would rise and perhaps even we can reverse the effects of menopause entirely. Let's just *think* ourselves pregnant and maybe it'll happen!

The problem with offering antidepressants as a *first step* is that it shifts the focus from your vagina to your mind – the wrong end of your body entirely. Of course it *may* be the case that you need to take antidepressants as well as other medication in order to help you maintain a normal and healthy mind, but to offer it instead of treatment to deal with the atrophy itself seems a little strange. It's almost as though we're making the condition up.

When I talk with other women who suffer from VA, they feel something similar: people assuming that they're '*just going through menopause*' and so are probably *just* feeling a bit blue. Nothing that a few pills can't sort out. It's sometimes because of this initial reaction from doctors, friends and family that women are feeling unable or unwilling to talk about their symptoms any further, worried that they'll get branded as '*menopausal*', as though that in some way explains away everything. Women are left feeling ashamed, isolated and, naturally, very depressed, not quite sure who to turn to or who will believe that they are in *physical* as well as *mental* pain.

I even experienced this myself.

Even though I've always been very open about my VA to my family, I couldn't help but feel like I was a burden to them, or that I was in some way exaggerating my pain. As much as my husband, daughters and son-in-laws gave me as much space as possible to talk about how I was or wasn't coping, I always had this niggling feeling that I should probably stop talking or that I should just say I was fine. I mean, who wants to talk about their mother's vagina anyway? Let alone their mother-in-law's! The sense of suffering can start to feel very isolating indeed.

I remember walking around the fields with Bertie and Bonnie one day and just sobbing my eyes out; crying heavy, painful tears and feeling deeply, deeply alone. The atrophy was unbearable, with every step making me feel like I was going to throw up. And the sense of loneliness was absolutely terrifying. On a rational level, I knew that I was loved dearly by my family but for some reason I couldn't really *feel* it. Even when I looked at my dogs I wondered whether they would even notice if I just slipped away gently, like a leaf down a stream. They'd adjust without me. They'd move on.

And so that's when I started to see a counsellor.

Counselling

Being in constant physical pain and not feeling able to really share the intricacies of it with friends and family, I was starting to feel very, very down. I've always been a very optimistic and practical person so this new sense of depression was a real shock to me; I now understand what people mean when they say they feel like they're being followed by a dark cloud all day. However sunny the day, or happy the occasion, for me it was always clouded with the pain of my vagina and vulva and the thought that my life would forever be like this. I was still very much in the early stages of finding a treatment and was getting desperate and disillusioned from the advice to *ignore it* or *have more sex* or that I *was fine*.

I wasn't fine.

By searching online, I managed to find this wonderful therapist who had been through menopause herself and now specialised in supporting other women through it, advocating for a more open and honest culture surrounding such issues. Once a fortnight for several months, I'd sit in her therapy room and just cry and cry and cry, not knowing what to do or how to make things better. I shared with her things I didn't want to tell my family and didn't feel guilty for bringing down the mood or ruining her day. Through these tears and honesty, I felt like I was beginning to cleanse myself from all the shame I had internalised from suffering with VA and felt truly listened to and supported. I wasn't judged. I wasn't seen as just another hysterical menopausal woman. I wasn't alone.

Through these sessions, I began to come to terms with living with chronic pain and began to practise the coping mechanisms my therapist recommended: meditation, body scanning, keeping a diary. At first I considered these to be a bit mumbo-jumbo, after all they didn't exactly deal with my atrophy, but with time they started to make more sense and I could incorporate them into my daily routine. I might not like vaginal atrophy but if I accepted it, maybe I could stop fighting it and free up some energy to find a treatment.

And so I surrendered to it.

I decided that enough was enough. The condition wasn't in my head. I wasn't going to feel dirty, or embarrassed or ashamed anymore. Just because we don't *like* talking about typically 'private' matters doesn't mean we shouldn't.

From this, I joined and set up online support groups, talking very frankly about VA and ridding the shame surrounding it. I could look at the medical professional in the eye and tell them that the advice for me to have sex and forget about it was inappropriate and misguided. I made an appearance on TV and radio about my own personal experiences and contributed to a menopause magazine with an article about my VA.

I've found a great deal of friendship within these online forums and tender care from the women who are also suffering. For me, these support groups and therapy sessions have been integral in my VA journey and I now try to dedicate as much time as I can to helping others. I walk between 3-5 miles everyday with my dogs to keep my mind clear and my body healthy and no matter how dark the days feel, I always try to go to bed remembering at least one ray of sunshine that found its way in.

~

Whilst I've now come to accept that vaginal atrophy is a chronic condition that will – literally, stay with me forever and will therefore never be 'cured', there are definitely things we can be doing and using to go at least *some* way to offer more permanent relief. Try oestrogen if you can. Visit your WHP. Consider laser treatment. Find products that suit you and establish a strict routine that helps your VA. Be kind to yourself and talk to a counsellor – it may help.

Don't accept that *this is it* or that *it's fine* or *'just'* meno-pause. Through the social sanitisation of 'The Change', I believe we've somehow come to accept that severe suffering in over half the population is normal, or acceptable, or unavoidable.

This is madness.

Though it *may* be the case that vaginal atrophy is a *common*, albeit horrific, consequence of ageing as a woman, I cannot understand how the medical and social understanding of it is still so primitive. Just today, a woman on my support group has been told to "accept it and move on", as though it were the common cold that caused a few inconvenient sniffles but would eventually clear up. Is it because we're not making enough fuss about vaginal atrophy that things aren't changing? If we all started actually revealing the true horror of vaginal dryness, would better treatment be found? Is it because of our silence that we're suffering so greatly from it?

If some of the medical advice I was given in 2018 was to have more sex when my vagina and vulva were so swollen, so red and so sore I could barely walk, there seems to be something very, very wrong with our understanding of the condition and of our treatment of women. I think until we all start talking openly about it, about the gruesome, gory and intimate details of vaginal atrophy, this expectation of silence and acceptance will only continue, leaving women all over the world feeling ashamed, alone and desperate. Would we give men the same advice if they went to the doctor with a swollen, bleeding and splitting penis? Would we *really* tell him to have more sex and to just forget about it? Or that it's a normal part of being a middle-aged man? I don't think so.

CHAPTER 7

Sex: Remember That?

Sex: it exhausts me just thinking about it!

I thought we were meant to be out of this mine-field when we were teenagers: *Are we getting it enough? When did we last do it? Is it meant to feel like that?* And yet now I seem to be thinking about it more than I ever have – but not of course in the same way.

My previous lust for 'It' has been replaced with fear. Questions between friends asking how many times a day do I *Do It* have been replaced with how many times a *year*. And the only penetration I seem to be getting is from a lubed-up, cabinet-stored plastic dilator which resembles more of a melted candle than a penis! No batteries, no sexy man, no orgasm. Just a flag pole stuck in the dry ground reminding me that, like the Queen, *She's* in residence – as though there was a chance I could somehow forget.

But when it comes to intimacy, I feel that sex is just one of those areas that simply *is* awkward to talk about. We want to seem normal, and healthy and attractive: not staying too close to the image of the Virgin Mary but not straying too far from it either. We're told to be sexy but not slutty, horny but still homely, experimental but not weird; that the length of our skirt or the dip of our neckline can determine whether we're a slut, a whore or a frigid bitch. It's no wonder that we find it tricky to talk about physical intimacy when our bodies can sometimes feel like they aren't wholly our own.

But if we saw menopause as a marker for sexual and physical liberation and as a recognition of our extraordinary femininity, I wonder whether we could go some way to change that: paying thanks and respects to our bodies if they have provided life, but then celebrating the freedom of future unbounded sexual exploration. No more condoms, no more pills, no more fear of unwanted pregnancies. Hooray!

And yet for many of us, at the time when sex should be so freeing and gloriously selfish, we feel instead constrained by the limitations of our bodies: we're left frustrated, just not sexually so. I often think that if I'd known my vagina would flake and ache as much as it does now, I'd probably have shagged with a bit more pizazz when I had the chance!

The problem, though, is that by its very nature sex is an activity that requires someone else. This can sometimes lead us to feeling responsible or obligated to fulfil another's sexual pleasure, even if it's to the detriment of our own.

When I first started experiencing vaginal dryness in my forties, I didn't think too much of it: lube it up, thumb it in and off you go. It wasn't until the discomfort and soreness became an everyday norm that I realised there was something more serious going on. Sex became more irregular, fading slowly at first and then one day falling sharply off the cliff-edge, leaving just an echo in my life.

So what was I to do: never make love to my husband again?

For months, I tried to persevere: using every lube available, from the organic massage oils to the moisturisers milked from the nipples of virgin angels. No matter how much it could slip and slide, I was always left feeling red-raw and fragile for days after. And yet when I finally plucked up the courage to speak to a doctor about it (not my own – she was away), I was told to simply have *more* sex: that if I continued to keep the runway closed, it was obvious that no plane would be able to land. No flight path, no holiday fun.

I was horrified. Perhaps I hadn't explained enough to them just how painful it was: how it felt like my episiotomies were tearing every time there was penetration; how I thought my vagina was going to prolapse; how I felt so alone and unattractive and utterly, utterly miserable.

But surely, in the same way that you can't land a plane in the middle of a blazing fire and expect to come out unscathed, so too can you not expect a woman to welcome a penis into her vagina when it's burning, thinning and splitting open: to do so would be madness, and abuse.

And yet, this is a reality for many thousands of women around the world. When I'm chatting to the women on my online support group, I'm constantly shocked at the number of them who are still having sex with their partners despite the pain and negative physical and emotional repercussions it's having on their bodies afterwards. Whilst many of them are having sex because *they* want to, notwithstanding the discomfort it causes, many are not: feeling obligated to satisfy their partners for fear of them leaving them or not fulfilling their sexual needs.

In many ways, whether that fear is normal or natural or justified or not is almost irrelevant: if we're enduring painful sex solely to serve the needs of someone else, I think we need to reevaluate our relationships and reflect on our own self-worth. Is our physical and mental well-being *really* second best to a quickie on a Friday night? Is it *really* our role as women to *serve* and *obey*? Will our partner *really* leave us if we cannot have sex with them anymore?

Maybe they will.

And if they do? Well, anyone who prioritises sex over soul simply isn't worth having in your life. You're better off on your own and you'll be OK.

I know of a woman who, after 40 years of marriage during which she raised four children and never had paid employment, was left going into retirement as a divorcee: no pension, no property, and no partner. Her husband had decided that he too had *needs* and that he couldn't face the final 20+ years of his life without any physical intimacy.

Now, who knows what problems there were in that relationship already, but what struck me most was the idea that intimacy=sex and that therefore no sex=no intimacy. I don't know about you but I've had some very disengaged, distant and disastrous sex in my life and similarly some of the most intimate moments have been when my husband tickles my back in the way he knows I like, or when he brings me a cup of tea in bed in the morning with just the right shade of brown, or when he holds my hand when I'm feeling sad. *Of course* we might want sex, it's a natural animal instinct and it's fun (!), but to promote it to a level higher than respect, support and friendship seems to be the wrong side of animalistic.

There are many ways to be intimate, and in fact one of the *most* effective ways to reach deep intimacy is trust. But to truly trust, we have to be honest, and that includes openness about our vaginal atrophy or menopause. How can we expect our partners to support us if we don't tell them what we're going through? If, once telling them, they don't support us, then it's for us to consider whether that is a relationship we want to continue.

And remember, ladies, there's so much more to sex than just *penis in vagina* (PIV) – it doesn't have to be all *in-out-*

in-out-shake-it-all-about. You shouldn't just give up on your sexual relationship with your partner just because you can't have penetrative sex. It's not an all-or-nothing thing and you definitely don't need to go the whole shebang to enjoy intimacy. Just think of those days when we were young and flirty and went all giggly and gooey when someone we fancied brushed past us in the corridor, or accidentally-on-purpose touched our hand when we were walking next to each other. Our vaginas would start to tingle just from the naughtiness of it all and we were still fully clothed! The intimacy came from the *desire* and the *secrecy* and the *suspense.* We need to try to cultivate that sense of fun and lightness again, even if it takes a bit of time.

So how can we be sexually intimate without penetration? Well, I'm sure you can answer this one as well as I can, but let's briefly consider our options. *But* because even I'm getting a bit out of my depth here, let's imagine sex as an ice-lolly. My son-in-law said this metaphor sounds a bit penis-y, and he's probably right, so try to imagine a non-phallic ice-lolly, if you will: one that encompasses vaginas, penises and nipples alike!

Of course, if we're feeling a bit hot and *really* want that ice-lolly, we can just gobble it all up in one – maybe getting brain freeze for eating it too fast but at least feel satisfied at the end. Fun, but maybe short-lived. But there are other ways we can eat that ice-lolly: we can suck it, lick it, nibble around the edges, wait for it to melt a bit beneath your hands. Even if you can't eat the whole ice-lolly, doesn't mean you can't have *some* of it and still enjoy it. In fact, sometimes, just having a little bit of something is nicer than having the lot – you appreciate it more, savour it a bit longer and think about how delicious it was and when you might next be able to try it again. It would be madness to think that you had to always eat the whole thing in order to be happy. The same goes with sex.

I know perhaps our generation (or maybe just me!) is much more sexually reserved than the next, but there really has been such a huge shift in sexual liberation that it's now totally up to you and your partner to set your own boundaries. There are no rules anymore. Sex doesn't just mean PIV. And sex toys *aren't* just for the kinky – they're for everyone! There have been big, big changes since the dawn of the Rampant Rabbit, and whilst that has done wonders for many women all over the world, it can perhaps also feel a bit threatening to older women, or women who are in pain and who aren't feeling all that sexy. And so whilst you might not want to use the fastest, biggest or most powerful vibrator there is, it doesn't mean you shouldn't at least *try* a sex toy (there are so many) to help you reach orgasm – after all, bringing blood flow back to the area, releasing endorphins and encouraging natural lubrication from the Bartholin glands, are all excellent ways to maintain good vaginal health. And you never know, you might even enjoy it!

I've signposted you to some excellent websites and sexual health experts who are much better at talking about all this than I am; go to the Acknowledgements at the back of the book to check out their details and have fun sexperimenting!

How to have sex (when *you* want to but your vagina doesn't)

But, practically, if we *do* want to have PIV sex what can we do to minimise the pain?

As well as moving away from popular chemical-heavy lubes, I started trying natural water or oil-based lubricants with varying levels of success. As we've already seen, using products that don't change the natural pH of our vaginas is hugely important in maintaining a healthy ecosystem, so please do bin those chemical heavy lubes and find something more natural. When I actually started researching all the things that are put into the more popular (and cheaper) lubricants, I was pretty horrified: I think I would have been kinder to my vagina if I'd just used the WD-40® in the shed (please don't try this at home). We *must* stop this insanity of putting poison into our bodies and pretending that it's normal. The only people it's helping are the big corporations selling the things! You wouldn't spray perfume onto a grazed knee so don't do the same with your genitals.

And in terms of sex, we have to remember that during menopause, because our oestrogen and testosterone levels can plummet, we're unlikely to be feeling all that sexually interested – this is because these hormones are essential for getting you in the mood and so if they're not there, your sex drive isn't likely to be there either. But for some women, once these hormones are replaced, they start to feel a bit flirty again, and yet for others menopause feels like a light switch: abruptly turning off any hint of libido.

On the other hand, some women also experience something known as the sex surge, where, like rabbits in the summer, they want to shag anything that moves. I've read some hilarious stories of husbands left almost cowering in the corner from too much sex (be careful what you wish for, eh?), petrified their rampant wives will want them again. This is due to our hormone imbalances and usually means our testosterone levels have surged higher than our bodies are used to. For some women, this surge can last a matter of days or weeks and for others this almost insatiable appetite for sex can last years. The problem of course, comes when you have the surge mentally but experience the soreness physically: the cruelty of never being able to scratch that itch.

For a while, I experienced this surge myself and felt really depressed about the thought of never being able to have sex again. In the meantime, however, I knew that if there was any chance of fitting a penis into my current pin-sized hole, I'd have to start work on expanding the area.

Dilators and vibrators

And so, upon buying a selection of the most sexually unstimulating dilators I could ever imagine, I took a Russian doll's approach to dilation: starting with the smallest and working my way up.

Now, of course, the purpose of these dilators isn't to aid sexual arousal but my goodness do they stop it! The first time I used it, my vagina seemed to turn into a stubborn toddler refusing food: clamped mouth, impressively strong jaw strength and never-demonstrated-before resilience. I had to almost do the whole "*Here comes the choo-choo train*" trick with my vagina to tempt the thing in. But eventually, and with tears and tantrums and *lots* of natural lube, I managed to work my way up to the size of a penis.

This took time and lots and lots of patience.

When I first bought the plastic dilators, the advice I was given was to start with the slimmest one – which was no wider than a finger – and then move onto the next size up *only* once the pain from using the smaller one had gone. And so, every night I'd take myself upstairs just before bed, lube up the dilator, find some rubbish on the internet to take my mind off what I was doing, take a deep breath and then on the exhale slowly push it in. I found that the biggest barrier to my pain was tensing up, and so after some breathing techniques, I was able to breathe my way through the discomfort more easily. The first attempt of course was very uncomfortable, reminding me of smear tests or when the doctors fiddle around in your bits when you're pregnant, like you're a Mary Poppins handbag.

After five minutes though, the pain would start to ease, and after 10 minutes I'd slowly take it back out, again on the exhale, and pat myself on the back for being so brave. I repeated this every night for 10 minutes and after about a fortnight would try the next size up, not pushing it if it hurt. I do wonder what little Bertie thought I was doing when he loyally followed me upstairs every night. Poor dog. The things he's seen!

But after moving onto the third size up, I felt like I'd reached a bit of a wall – the level of discomfort just didn't go away and I started to feel miserable. It was then that a friend reached out to me and sent me a vibrator to try instead, claiming that the softer and more natural-feeling material would help to relax me and wouldn't feel as hard or as abrasive on my sensitive skin and sore vagina.

What a godsend! It really did help.

For me, I couldn't and didn't want to use it with batteries because my skin was already hypersensitive and I didn't want to risk it causing me more damage to the thinning skin around my vulva, but I know of ladies who use it as a normal vibrator and feel like they've got their old sex drive back. And as we've just read, orgasms are actually really *good* for us, not just psychologically but physiologically too. As well as releasing tension and anxiety, having sex and reaching orgasm also helps to keep our vaginal tissues well lubricated by bringing blood flow to the area. If we *can* reach orgasm, it might actually *help* our atrophy. But of course, for many of us, this feels like a bit of a cruel twist of fate: our atrophy is so bad that we can no longer have sex but we know that sex might perhaps help it. So that's why dilators and vibrators are great at helping us out while we can't have intercourse. And yet many women I know would simply never entertain the idea of using it, even for medical reasons, for fear of upsetting their partners or feeling that they're not the 'type' to use a sex toy. But if you look at some of the websites at the back of the book, you'll see that some sex toys these days look so inconspicuous and elegant you could almost put them on your dresser as an ornament!

And I do wish there wasn't still such a stigma around sex and orgasms with respect to women. It seems part and parcel of being a man that he'll masturbate throughout his life and that it's normal and healthy and expected, indeed perhaps even *worrying* if he never did. For women, on the other hand, there's still this feeling of desperation and vulgarity to it; that if a woman wants to pleasure herself sexually she's somehow commenting on her partner's inability to fulfil her, or more, that she's insatiable or some new-age man-hating feminist. From the conversations I have with my daughters though and from what I can see being sold to the next generation, I think this is changing for our younger women who seem to be more sexually liberated and confident. I'm pleased for them and hope this continues. But from what I hear about on my online support groups, thousands of women my age still have this sense of sexual duty to their partner or this mentality that seeking out your own sexual pleasure is in some way dirty. Even if they think the dilators and vibrators might actually help them with having a normal sex life again, they still refuse to use them because of the stigma surrounding them. I hope one day we're free of this repression.

And so, after those months of stretching and flexing my vagina, I did try to have sex again – very cautiously, very tentatively, very unattractively – and I was pleased to see that I could. Of course, I didn't orgasm, but that wasn't the point of my first attempt: I wanted to see whether, through care and time, my body could go some way to mending itself. I am still very much on that journey.

What I am pleased I didn't do, was to follow the advice I was given at the start of my VA journey and have sex anyway, forcing a penis into my body when it was clearly in distress and in need of TLC. We wouldn't walk on a broken leg, or poke a nasty bruise; we shouldn't do the same with our vaginas if they're sore, or irritated or painful.

You and your partner

But, of course, had I not been married to such a non-judgmental and supportive husband, I might have gone down the route of many of the women I've spoken to, and just put up with the pain of sex anyway – feeling I had no other option.

I ask you women to please talk to your partners if you're in pain and need to stop having sex. Let's not expect so little of our partners that we don't give them the opportunity to handle the truth. But similarly, let's not respect ourselves so little that we continue to endure pain even if they can't. I can't imagine any cultural, religious, biological or social reasoning that would ever convince me that one person has a *right* to have sex with you.

What I think we *do* need to do however, is to have a very frank and honest conversation with our partners, understanding that vaginal atrophy *does* affect them also. They too are likely to be feeling very isolated and unattractive and helpless, not knowing what to do to make you better, or wondering what your relationship will become if you can never express yourself sexually with each other again. That's tough.

When I eventually plucked up the courage to deal with the lack of sex in our marriage openly, I was saddened to hear that my husband had actually been feeling pretty awful: thinking that I wasn't attracted to him anymore, feeling guilty and ashamed for wanting to have the very physical

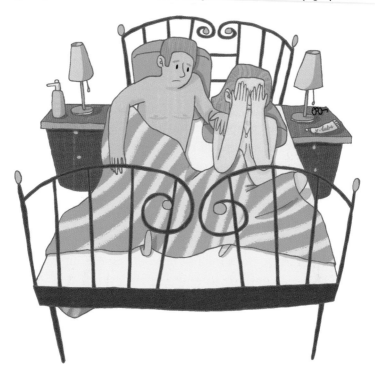

intimacy that he knew would hurt me, and then remembering our younger days with bouncy boobs and balls and debauchery. He was sad and, like me, longed for a time when we were fit and fiery.

It was when he reminded me of our younger days together that I realised just how much the haziness of constant pain had affected me. I had forgotten that we'd once actually had a healthy and happy and fun sex life, desiring each other physically and enjoying the pleasure our bodies could give each other. I didn't realise he was mourning that era of our life together, when we were sexy and spirited. Since VA, the relationship with my body, especially my vagina, had become so negative I had totally lost any concept of sexiness about it: I didn't feel attractive or confident in my body at all. My pubes were grey and thinning, my wobbly bits had taken on a whole new rhythm, and no matter what position I sat, lay or stood in, I felt like a red-hot poker had been stuck up my bits and was searing me from the inside out. The thought of another red-hot poker coming towards me was just too much! My husband has always been so kind and patient and non-judgemental and has never made me feel like I have to do anything I don't want to. He's comforted me when I've been left feeling angry and frustrated in bed and has still tried to make me feel beautiful. I'm very lucky.

But in the mean-time, if you've tried the ice-lolly metaphor but still aren't all that sure what to do with your partner, what else can you be doing to show physical intimacy if you can't have sex?

Well, what about a massage? Taking the time to actually tend to each other's tired and aching bodies I think is a pretty intimate way of expressing love and care – and it feels great too so would go some way to satisfy that want for physical contact. Why not take each other on a date, or make dinner with each other with some music on, or just watch a film together on the sofa wrapped in blankets? I know of women who have started dance classes, language lessons, walking clubs with their partners or have taken up new skills together like painting, cooking or playing a musical instrument, all with the view of making time and space for each other during a period when they might be feeling otherwise isolated. My husband and I try to go for walks together and explore different local woods or fields – sometimes taking a picnic or just sitting on a bench holding hands. You could even do what one couple did and buy a potter's wheel, recreating that scene from Ghost with Patrick Swayze and Demi Moore – now, if *that* isn't sexy, I don't know what is!

But there is a reality that we also need to accept: for some people, sex is *very* important and no matter how much pottery porn we do, it simply won't replace the real thing. And that's where an honest conversation comes in with your partner *accepting* that they might still be wanting to have sex, or something close to it, and exploring how they might be able to achieve that in a way that you both feel comfortable with.

Encourage your horny husband to take his left hand on a date in the shower, or massage him with a little bit more swag in the areas he might enjoy. The same goes for your wives or girlfriends. Some women load up some 'naughty' images or videos online and give their partner's a helping hand to reach climax so that they still feel like they're part of the process. Whatever works for you! Just, for goodness sake, don't keep having sex if it's hurting you; there's no fun in that, and I'm sure if your partner found out the reality of

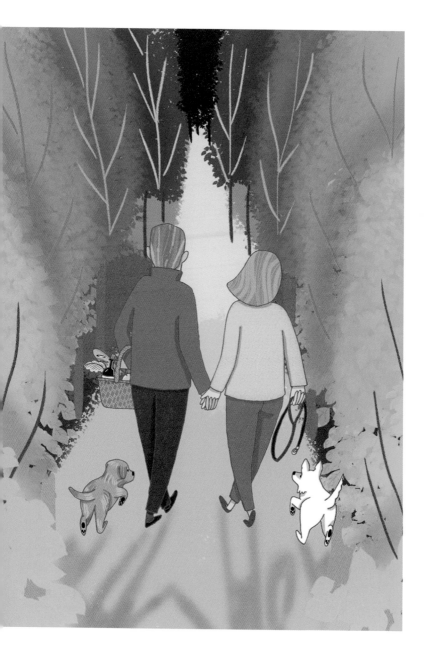

your pain they'd be horrified. If they're not, then *you* should be horrified.

So in the meantime, whether you want to have sex or not, try using dilators or vibrators in order to bring back blood flow to the area and keep your vagina hydrated. Be gentle with yourself and start with the slimmest first, using lots of natural lube, and work your way up. If your clitoris isn't painful, try using a vibrator to help you reach orgasm but if it is, perhaps distract yourself by watching TV, listening to a meditation podcast, or reading a book. Take advantage of all the discreet and luxurious sex toys out there. Be kind to yourself and be honest with your partner – encourage them to be honest with you too.

Sex is to be enjoyed, not endured. My son-in-law once sent me a picture of one of those plaques you see on a park bench that's been dedicated to a lost loved one. It read: "In loving memory of my darling wife, *If it isn't fun, don't do it!*"

I couldn't have said it better myself.

CHAPTER 8

Friends and Family

One of the biggest successes of my online support group has been providing women with a community to talk openly about their issues, worries and experiences. We all know that suffering in silence only makes the problem worse and by keeping everything quiet we're not only damaging ourselves but are also potentially harming our daughters, granddaughters, families and friends, perpetuating future suffering. You won't believe the amount of times I've had a cup of tea with a woman who has sighed in relief when I started describing my own experiences so that she too could now talk about her burning vagina without feeling embarrassed. My daughters too often come to me with a story about one of their friends or friend's family who are suffering from vaginal pain, and when they're directed my way, they often feel a relief that it isn't only them.

Woman to woman

Sometimes the irony in life is that those we love and support the most are also the ones who can hurt us the deepest. This is why families are often so disastrously chaotic. The same goes for sisterhood.

What I think has hurt me the most along this journey, other than the actual atrophy, have been the times when I've either been ignored, ridiculed or actively berated.

This is true even more so when it's been with women I was confiding in.

I remember when I first 'confessed' to a female friend about my physical struggle: the look of discomfort, unease and disgust, was really hurtful. I know now that it was probably a reflection of her own inability to handle difficult situations, rather than the palatability of the condition itself but it taught me a great deal about the human tendency to avoid unpleasant or uncomfortable circumstances.

No matter what, we must talk openly with each other. Yes, it's awkward. Yes, it's embarrassing. No, you might not want to talk about your drying vagina over a plate of spag bol with your boss, but the fact is: you should talk about it. And around your children – both girls and boys. Have difficult conversations about intimate areas and watch the relief on their faces when they realise they don't have to be ashamed. Feeling shame is a learned behaviour: make sure you aren't teaching it in your household or modelling it in friendship groups.

Even in online *support* forums I've witnessed some unkindness between women, some of them suggesting that the other is exaggerating or that her pain isn't as worthy or as bad as theirs. This is madness.

What is more maddening is that, even on my own forum (having been set up by a woman, for women, with the highest privacy settings available) I still encounter women who are too embarrassed to post their problems in the group. They may watch conversations between other members, gathering information, feeling less alone, but then will message me privately asking about some condition or symptom they are dealing with. How can we fight this battle if, even behind closed doors and in a safe community, women are feeling so ashamed of speaking out that they can't even do it amongst fellow sufferers?

Don't be one of these women, however shy or embarrassed you feel. Listen to your friend. But most importantly, be an agent for change and start the conversation. Listen to your mum, your daughter, your neighbour or annoying colleague. Open up about your own experiences and let them know that you'll support them, that they're not alone. When you feel yourself judging them because they're handling the condition in a different way to you, stop yourself and remember that we're all on different journeys and that we're all getting on with it in the best way we know how.

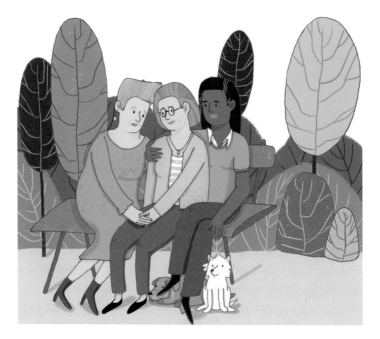

Woman to partner

I'm lucky. My husband has been an absolute dream through this nightmare and has suffered every ache, pain, anguish and every tear I've shed along with me. He has brought me frozen baked beans cans to cool my vulva down, hot water bottles to heat it back up, and watched me insert every type and size of dilator, gloop and gel in the place that used to give us both joy. He has taken more pictures of my vulva than I think he ever has of my face in our 34 years of marriage and he's never once made me feel ugly, or embarrassed, guilty or ashamed.

But I know that this isn't the case for every woman.

Many women I've encountered find the lack of understanding in their relationship as hard as, or if not harder than, the physical problems themselves. I'm truly horrified by the number of women who are continuing to have sex despite being in absolute agony. I don't care whether you think the obligation to have sex is a cultural, religious, contractual, emotional or physical need, I object to it 100% if it causes you distress. And if you think your partner wouldn't understand or that they have certain *needs* that must be fulfilled, I think it's important to take the time to consider just how healthy that relationship really is. Would you want your daughter putting up with that?

Of course, when I stopped having sex with my husband I felt a whole plethora of emotions: guilt, sadness, disgust, anxiety, fear, worry. Would he still love me? Would he want to go off and have sex with other women? Should I let him? Was I ruining his life as well as my own? I worried that I was making a fuss, that I was letting him down as a wife and that I should just *lie back and think of England* whether I liked it or not.

I think, as women, we're used to putting others before ourselves and it can sometimes feel like we're being selfish if we prioritise our own needs.

We need to get better at that.

But depending on the type of relationship you have with your partner, it might be really difficult to be open and honest about the impact the menopause is having on your vagina or vulva. There may be many reasons for this: your partner might not be emotionally available to have such a conversation; it might be culturally taboo to speak so brazenly about such matters; they simply may not have experience in talking about women's health issues. I'm sure we all know of the brothers, dads, friends who would shy away even from 'period talk' growing up, or of the male teachers who would whimper in terror and let you leave a lesson if you told them you were on your period. If we're not teaching our boys how to talk maturely about women's matters, I'm not sure to what extent we can expect our men to be any better. If we create a culture within our own homes, and within our own relationships, that perpetuates that secrecy, then we're going to find it harder to speak publicly about private matters when we need to.

So, irrespective of the reason why you've not been able to discuss your vaginal atrophy with your partner, make a change today and speak out to them. We shouldn't feel ashamed of a condition that a) isn't your fault, b) is impacting significantly on your quality of life and c) will potentially be experienced by over half the world's population in some degree. Perhaps give your partner this book, so they can find out about the issues you're facing without you having to talk directly about it. If you don't open up about what you're going through, you can't expect them to understand or help you.

Let them know that sex is hurting and that you would love to be intimate with them in other ways, but that at the moment you can't have intercourse. There are many ways to be loving and to fulfil our desires for physical intimacy: give them a massage, sit together on the sofa and watch a film, hold hands when you're talking to each other. For me, a healthy relationship isn't built on a one-sided orgasm; it's built on mutual respect, honesty and the willingness to adapt to and comfort each other as we grow older.

Mother to daughter

This book isn't designed to scare our daughters – quite the opposite. I hope it will empower them. If we can go throughout our lives knowing which signposts to follow when we come across an unknown path, or that we're not alone in our time of need, then there's hope.

We're all told from an early age to check our breasts for lumps and know to go to the doctor if we find one, the same should be practiced for our vaginas and vulvas.

Again, we must remember that shame is a learned behaviour; something we're taught. My 3-year old granddaughter doesn't feel embarrassed about walking around the house naked, or going for a wee in front of us and this is because my daughter does the same around her.

We must set the right example for them: have a bath with them and let them see your squishy and hairy bits; get dressed with them so they can see the difference between mummy in Spanx® and mummy without; show them your sanitary towel when they're staring at you on the loo so they understand what menstrual blood looks like.

How many of you grimaced at the last sentence? And why is that?

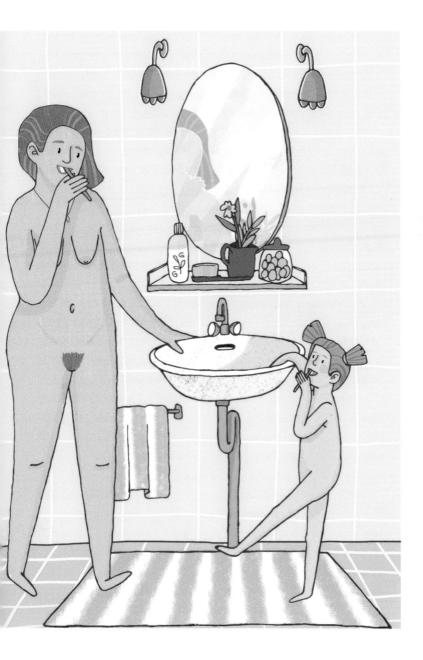

Because it's a 'private' matter? Because they're 'too young' to understand? Because it's dirty? It's something that will happen to them; something that we cannot control; and something that they shouldn't be ashamed of. In fact, that's the very reason why *Samaritans* was first set up; in 1953, a 14 year old girl started her period and because no one had ever told her it was a natural process of growing up, she killed herself. Even when I started my period at just 10 years old, I knew very little about it. I remember feeling really scared about what was happening to me and trying to hide it desperately from everyone around. Fast forward 40 years and that tendency to hide away and feel ashamed seems to have followed me and many other women I talk with. I don't want that for my daughters and granddaughters.

As a society we seem to be pretty squeamish about the undressed body and I suspect this plays a significant factor in the way we view ourselves as we grow up. My daughter is a teacher and she's constantly dealing with young people who are dieting, or who are already obsessed with going to the gym, or who are negatively concerned about their body image. Girls come to her embarrassed about having to go to the toilet during lessons to change their sanitary towels and often skip P.E so their peers can't see them in their underwear when they're getting changed.

How is this still happening? Why are our children still feeling so much shame? When will we stop being embarrassed about being women?

And yet in many ways, in the UK there hasn't been a better time to be a woman, with many movements focusing directly on addressing equality and *equity* between genders: the *#MeToo* international movement against sexual assault and harassment; the *Everyday Sexism Project* that exposes the daily sexism against women that has become almost normalised in our society; the *Sling the Mesh* campaign that brings awareness to the suffering of so many women who have undergone vaginal mesh surgery.

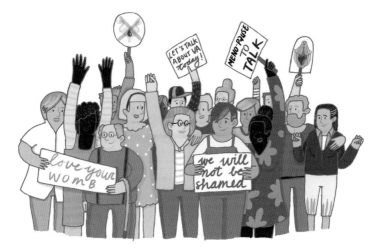

We are finally seeing that women everywhere are no longer willing to keep quiet. We have a voice and we want it heard.

Women are moving into all areas of society that had once been the sole domain of men – and they're getting there by merit. Recently, my son-in-law took great delight in hearing, for the first time, a woman commentating on, not just any football match, but the World Cup. Can you imagine how that would have gone down even a few years ago? These doors for women didn't open by themselves: they've been banged on and hacked down by generations of women previously. We owe it to them to continue.

Indeed, as the first female statue ever erected in Parliament Square, I think suffragist Millicent Fawcett would be pretty happy to see our *second* female Prime Minister sitting in the most powerful chair in the country. Irrespective of your political persuasion, this is progress. But even as Fawcett stands there ever-determined, we still have much to learn from the words inscribed on her banner: "*Courage calls to courage everywhere.*"

We must be more courageous as women. We must question inherited social norms and get rid of the ones that don't serve us. We must be brave with our children and teach them not to be ashamed of their bodies.

Let's start a new dialogue with our girls and begin by teaching them the correct words for their genitals. Let's empower them and talk to them about how it might feel during puberty, and what will happen during their first period, and how it might hurt the first time they have sex. Let's discuss how we're coping with menopause and how we're surprised about what's happening and how it can feel a bit isolating and lonely at times.

Let's be honest.

Mother to son

And the same goes for our sons, of course.

I'm very lucky with my son-in-laws as their strong wives and girlfriends have given them no choice but to enter the Vagina Dialogue. On any given day they might text me asking "*How's your vag, Jane?*" followed usually by an emoji of a fire and a silly face to symbolise both the burning and the peculiarity of the conversation. Though this conversation sometimes feels strange, wrong even, ultimately, I'm proud.

I'm proud that my daughters are strong women. I'm proud that their partners are strong men. I'm proud that they're looking out for me and that they're not allowing me to cope with this on my own.

They know that I can't have sex anymore and so they're aware that one day that might be true of their own wives, my daughters. Or it might not. But what they now know is that sex *can* be a problem and so an ongoing conversation needs to be had about it. They understand about the importance of regular health checks and personal examinations of both their own and their partner's genitals. They're not ashamed to talk about body parts that are usually hidden away from society and nor do they feel the shame of discussing irregularities with their own bodies if they notice something. They understand that women's health is a man's issue too; whether it's their partner, sister, aunt, mum, daughter, colleague or friend, they're prepared to have a conversation that is often avoided to show that they're there to support without judgement.

With this unusually in-depth knowledge about the many characteristics and personalities of a vagina, they also know that sex can be far from enjoyable and so I hope they'll be better equipped to look out for my daughters when I no longer can.

Of course, this situation is probably highly unusual; I'm not sure how many other mother and son-in-law relationships talk so openly about vaginas, let alone their own, so I'm not professing for you all to start texting your relatives about your *ring of fire*, unless you want to! But I think we should give our sons and son-in-laws more credit; they're probably able to deal with the topic better than we think. And if they aren't? Well, it's never too late to learn.

CHAPTER 9

A Final Thought

So why the lack of education?

If any of what I've written has been a surprise to you, you're not alone. It was for me too. It wasn't until I started perimenopause that I even considered that my vagina would age. Each month I'd see my face sag and my boobs drop, my skin sallow and my wrinkles deepen, but I'd give no thought to my vagina. Now, I feel like such a fool – of course if my skin was drying and ageing, my vagina and vulva would be too. Why didn't I know that?

And I think that's an important question. Why don't we know vital and, ultimately, life-changing information about our own bodies? About what to expect, how to manage it and how long it will last? I was aware that my vagina would bleed every month, would discharge, would probably tear and be sewn back up during child birth: I might not have liked the prospect, but at least I felt prepared. But for the burning? The constant soreness and irritation? The hyper-sensitivity to every fabric, surface and temperature? The inability to have sex with my husband? No, I was not prepared for that. I was not prepared to deal with this much pain in my later years. And according to my support groups, I wasn't the only one.

It seems that the words *vaginal atrophy* have somehow escaped our vocabulary, and even when they do eventually find their way to our lips we seem able only to whisper them in embarrassment, shame or confusion. How many people know about *your* vaginal atrophy? Have you discussed it with friends, family or colleagues? Have you even admitted to yourself that VA might be what you have?

Though I wouldn't exactly describe my physical situation as *fortunate*, in many ways I do feel lucky with the support I've had in dealing with my VA. Now I feel able to speak openly about my experiences with my family and I never feel that I've had to handle it all on my own. Take this book as an example – it's been a real family effort: whether it was writing the actual words, editing the content or proof-reading the many, many drafts, it has been my family who have helped make this happen and their support and encouragement has been invaluable in my journey.

My vagina has travelled the world, pinging between email accounts from London to Northamptonshire, New Zealand to China, every email helping out to get my story shared so that others don't feel alone. Many a Skype chat has been centred around my oestrogen routine, (lack of) sex life, or my greying pubes; conversations I would never have imagined having seven years ago, are now spoken freely between generations over a cup of tea or a bowl of cereal.

I know that without the unwavering support from my family I wouldn't be as strong as I am today. I can honestly say there hasn't been a single nook or cranny of my anatomy that hasn't been spoken about in depth round the dinner table. My daughter said a funny thing the other day that I think sums up the last few years: "*I think my husband has spent more time with your vagina, Mum, than mine!*" Whilst this is a strange image for a mother to have, I couldn't help but laugh when she said this.

But rather than feel sad, or embarrassed, or guilty about that, I feel strong. Not strong for me, though, strong for *them*. Strong for my girls: my three beautiful daughters and my precious little granddaughter. By speaking up about my vaginal atrophy I hope I've gone some way to bring down the barriers for them, should they ever need the support. Whatever happens in my life, I will feel that little bit happier knowing that my girls (and the men they've chosen to walk by their sides) are better equipped to handle their changing bodies than I was.

And I guess, perhaps selfishly, I feel that my daughters know what to look out for when I'm old and frail and may be too weak to fight my own battles. Because anyone who's ever been in constant pain will know just how exhausting it is and how much physical and mental strength you need just to get through one day. It is no exaggeration that my VA journey has been a full-time job: researching how and why women get it; looking for ways to stop the pain; finding medical professionals knowledgeable and willing enough to help.

I hope that having read this book you will feel that there is not only hope, but a myriad of products, therapies, and routines that you can try which can go some way to improving your quality of life. But I also hope you have discovered that the first and most critical step, is opening up (about) your vagina!

It is so important that we first start talking about VA if we are ever going to get the help, love, care and support we need. Though none of us ever really knows what the future holds, I know I share a common fear amongst women with VA, that I'll end up in a situation where I'm in immense pain but am somehow unable to communicate it properly.

Who will apply my oestrogen gel and moisturisers then? Who will help me research new creams and treatments when the ones I'm currently using stop working?

Knowing that my daughters have the knowledge to help me, gives me at least some comfort as I go into old age; I've basically told them, if in doubt, just to squirt oestrogen into every orifice until I bubble over! Smuggle it in and shove it up!

I was horrified the other day when my friend, who works in a nursing home, told me that none of the elderly women under her care are given oestrogen: no creams, gels or patches for any of them. In fact, as far as she could tell, there's no provision for menopausal symptoms at all, other than the occasional blow-up cushion to ease the discomfort of a sore bum. It is truly horrifying to imagine all the countless women the world over who are sitting alone in their rooms with unimaginable pain between their legs and no way of getting help.

How many of you have mothers, grandmothers, aunties, friends in a nursing home? How many of them do you know suffer from VA? How many of them do you know are getting help? Have you ever asked them?

The process of writing this book has been another milestone in helping me come to terms with my VA. Flicking through the pages I can see clearly the progress I've made through sheer bloody mindedness and a refusal to give up. There really are lots of ways that you can get help, and I hope having made it to the end of this book you feel empowered to seek help in the right places, from the right people and in the right way. Please continue reading to the very end as there are many products and experts I've listed that might be of help. You don't need to suffer in silence. There are millions of women out there who are experiencing issues just like you, make contact with some of them. They are your greatest friends and your biggest support network: you just haven't met them yet. The support I've received and been able to give has played a huge part in keeping my spirit alive while the oils, creams, therapies and doctors worked on my body. I am hopeful for the future and you should be too. Women's health has never looked so good. With your help, we can continue to make it better.

So ladies, my final plea to you is to educate yourselves, your family and your friends, males and females alike, so that you can help and support each other. Learn about your anatomy! Have a look at yourself in the mirror so you can spot changes and irregularities. Talk about your issues openly with the people closest to you. Now that I've shared my story, I hope you will share yours. It is no longer OK to 'keep quiet, shut up and put up' with this pain, like our fore-mothers did. We will not be shamed. We'll be kind to each other, to our vaginas and our vulvas. We'll speak up, seek help and be strong because we love and care for ourselves, and because we love and care for our friends, sisters, daughters and granddaughters.

And by gathering the strength of all the incredibly brave and inspiring women who went before us, we'll do all that we can to make women's lives better everywhere, never judging each other, never belittling the suffering of others. We'll think of Millicent Fawcett as she stands stoically in Parliament Square, the only woman among the monuments, and we'll heed the advice written on her banner:

"Courage calls to courage everywhere."

Take courage.

Helpful Things

Products I like

I really ummed and ahhed about including this section in the book for fear of you thinking I was just trying to push products or that I had an affiliation with certain companies. In the end, though, I decided to put it in anyway because I know how desperate I was when I needed some relief and how grateful I would've been if someone had pointed me in the right direction.

Before I tell you what products have worked for me, I want to just make a few things clear:

- I've received absolutely no money from any of these companies.

- None of these companies have approached me to include their product in this book.

- You should always try the products yourself before incorporating them into a daily routine.

Moisturisers and oils

I've tried a *lot* of different oils, moisturisers and gels all professing to help menopausal women with their drying vaginas and vulvas. Unfortunately, with the majority of these products I had to throw them away after one application because I developed an allergic reaction or my skin became very sensitive to it. When I researched the ingredients contained within them, I was pretty shocked at what I found: perfumes, strange chemicals, unnecessary fillers. What I realised then, was that my body needed to have only natural ingredients put onto and into it so that it was soothed *naturally*. From my own experiences, I found the ones below to be the best for my skin type.

Olive and Bee

This moisturiser is branded as an *Intimate Cream* and was created by an Australian women's health physiotherapist relatively recently. As the name suggests, it's 100% natural and contains only olive oil and beeswax.

I use Olive and Bee as my moisturiser in the vestibule area and on my perineum twice daily (or as necessary). I like that it doesn't contain any nasty chemicals and is easy to throw into my bag when I'm out and about. For me, this is a staple.

Emuaid

Emu oil may not be suitable for the vegans or vegetarians out there as it's taken from the byproduct (fat) of the emu bird. Before you skip this option though, please do take a moment to do your own research on it as I've found from my support group that this is actually the product that ladies seem to get on with really well.

Basically, the antioxidant levels found in emu oil allows it to penetrate the skin deeply and helps ease the irritation from vaginal atrophy symptoms. It can be quite effective at calming the burn or easing the soreness if you suffer from it.

But please make sure you're buying the best emu oil you can because some of them have added chemicals to bulk them out. Like most things in life, you usually get what you pay for!

I use a product called Emuaid in the same way as Olive and Bee and V Magic below – I apply it to any area of my vulva that is dry, itchy or sore. My daughter even thinks it sorted out a particularly glowing spot she had on her face, so you can probably use this oil for a whole multitude of things.

V Magic

This is another moisturiser that contains only natural ingredients (six in total) and acts as a great daily cream to lubricate your vulva or any area of dryness. I use this in rotation with the other two external moisturisers above to ensure my skin doesn't become too sensitised to one product.

Yes!

This company has a range of different products that are based in either water or oil. They also have a vaginal moisturiser that you insert into the vagina through an applicator: you can either buy a large bottle and withdraw small amounts through a syringe each time, or buy individual ones where you snap off the top and dispose of the tube each time you've used it. It's really convenient for trips away, or to have in your handbag when you're on the move. I use this vaginal moisturiser every other night in rotation with local oestrogen – rather than using the individual ones, I use the syringe and applicator as it's not only cheaper but it's better for the planet as it produces less plastic waste.

Unlike Olive and Bee and V Magic, *Yes!* is an *internal* moisturiser and helps to moisten the vagina. I use this in combination with the external moisturisers to try to keep both my vulva and vagina moisturised and lubricated.

Yes! also offer a range of natural lubricants for sex and fore-play, so do have a browse of all their products to see if there's anything that might help you – I really like them.

Meditation apps

When I first started seeing a counsellor, she mentioned that I should try to find some time to meditate in whatever way I found comfortable. For me, walking with my dogs has always been my meditation but I know of many women who would really benefit from an app they could use on their way to work or when they're trying to get to sleep that helps them to cope with their pain. If I were a more dedicated meditator I would probably really like the apps called *Calm* and *Headspace*; both offer loads of short guided meditations that deal with anxiety, depression and living with pain. The *Calm* app also has a section called *Masterclasses* where people give a lecture on how to best live a mentally and physically good life. My daughter and son-in-law swear by them.

Sanitary products

It's pretty horrific the things they put in sanitary products these days. If you open up a clean sanitary towel or tampon and it smells quite nice or floral, then it's probably got per-fume or a nasty chemical in it that could irritate your vulva. Though all my life I had just used the normal sanitary prod-ucts like everyone else, when I hit perimenopause I found them to be incredibly uncomfortable causing me to sweat and itch from the irritation of the chemicals. I found some organic towels in the supermarket but they weren't very well-shaped and they didn't exactly cater for women who had heavy periods. And so I went searching online and found a product that I now use all the time: TOTM.

TOTM stands for *Time of the Month* and they offer all sanitary products delivered directly to your door. On their website, they claim to be '*100% organic, cruelty-free, biodegradable tampons, pads and liners*' and don't put any nasty chemicals into their products. From the first time I used them, the itching and irritation I started to experience from the other ones stopped entirely and I was able to go throughout a whole period without having any problems to my skin. Now even my daughters use them and have them delivered to their doors. Whilst they are definitely more expensive than more popular brands, if like me your atrophy caused extreme soreness to your vulva skin, they'll definitely be worth it.

Seat cushion

I'm afraid I've become one of those women who takes a cushion around with them rather than a handbag, throwing it down on every train, cinema or bench seat I sit on. I bought the orthopaedic cushion sold by SmithHillman as it's memory foam and sounded like it would provide me proper support. I love it – it means I can sit on the grass with my granddaughter and have a picnic or watch a film with my family. I prefer the medium-firm cushion but I know they also offer a firmer one, so I guess it's personal choice. I got mine from **www.smithhillman.co.uk**

Acknowledgements

I can't believe we've just written a book about my vagina! That's not normal, is it? I'm both delighted and terrified by finally finishing this little project; whilst I really hope that I've at least helped a few people along the way, I'm pretty nervous about having exposed myself so greatly. My intention though has always been to help.

Firstly, I really want to thank *you* for reading this book. If we can have as many people reading about vaginal atrophy as possible I am confident that better treatment will eventually be available to suffering women. By exposing the reality of VA, something better *will* be done about it, I am sure.

To all the thousands of women on my online support groups who have helped me *every day*, you are absolute saints and have saved me over and over again. I thank you from the bottom of my heart for not judging me. I couldn't have got to where I am today without you all. Stay strong. Keep going. Together we can do this.

And in alphabetical order (because I spent too long stressing about which order to thank you all in), I'd like to give an enormous thank you to the following extraordinary women who are going above and beyond to raise the profile for women's mental and physical wellbeing:

Thank you so much to Diane Danzebrink for being the most calming and kind therapist I could have wished for and for always making me feel like I had someone to turn to. You empowered me and gave me hope. In fact, it's because of you that this book first got kicked into action. I'd recommend for everyone to check out Diane's wealth of knowledge and expertise at http://menopausesupport. co.uk. Thank you, Diane for looking out for women's mental health at a time when they need it the most.

To Sam Evans aka Jo Divine, it's so great to see another woman so unafraid of talking about vaginas and vulvas! Thank you so much for dedicating your time to the liberation of women and the education of society in respect of sex: for reminding us that sex isn't just about PIV, and that intimacy can be found in all sorts of places, not just in our pants! Please all check out her incredible products and information pages at http://www.jodivine.com

To Fiona Mitchell, my wonderful women's health physiotherapist, who has always put me at ease and made me feel like there was hope – thank you for your continued patience, kind manner and support in my journey, I really appreciate everything you've done for me. To anyone looking for a WHP of their own, you'd do very well to have Fiona on your side https://www.harbornephysio.co.uk

Thank you Dr Louise Newson for your invaluable input into the first drafts of this book and for your ever encouraging words and support, your kind comments really uplifted me when I was having doubts about the book and your commitment to women's health more generally is inspiring. I have learnt so much from https://menopausedoctor.co.uk and greatly look forward to hearing about the successes of the Newson Health Menopause & Wellbeing Clinic in Stratford-upon-Avon, may this be the first of many.

To Amanda Tozer, sorry for farting in your face that time but thank you so much for laughing about it and never making me feel silly or embarrassed! It was so refreshing to find you: you are so down to earth, have a great sense of humour, and felt like you really cared about me at a time when I felt so low – thank you for giving me a hug when I cried. I would really recommend everyone checking out http://www.amandatozer.com

To Julie Bennett, there are simply no words to describe how grateful we are for the time and effort you have put into this book. Even when you were not feeling well yourself, you pulled out all the stops (and coffee pots) to help us out. Your knowledge and skill was invaluable in editing, as was your ability to break my hyphen obsession in a way that made me laugh. Thank you so much for all that you have done, we are eternally grateful.

I'd like to thank a few people more generally for their support, non-judgment and encouragement in writing this book: Dr Duncan, Jolien Kempen at studiostunner.com, Sabhbh Curran, Rhiannon Williams, Liam D'Arcy-Brown and Rebecca Probert – whether it was from publishing advice, proof-reading help or illustration skills, without your input the book wouldn't be what it is.

And finally to my family. It's no word of a lie when I say I couldn't have written this on my own. Thank you Penny for finding the time between teaching, having migraines and moving to China to co-write this book. It wouldn't have been written without you. I know this might not have been your intended first book title, but at least you achieved your goal of writing a book before you were 30! Thank you George for being brutally honest in your edits: although it was painful at times, it was necessary and very helpful.

You have done more than your fair share of writing and editing the book and I am very grateful for all the support you give me, including when you text me to find out how my vag is.

Gina, I am so proud of the mother you have become and of the beautiful daughter you have raised in Evie. It sometimes takes my breath away how you manage to fit in everything you do and still find the time to make sure I'm OK. Thank you for all your love, support and kind-hands. You cannot imagine how happy it makes me seeing my daughter bring up her own daughter so well.

Thank you Sam for your constant love and support, even though you are so far away. Your generosity and thoughtfulness never goes unnoticed and we are incredibly proud of everything you have achieved – it sounds like you've got a little piece of Home Farm and Gran in your New Zealand paradise and it makes us very happy to know you've got such a kind husband as Andrew to share it all with you, even if he does have rabbit eyes when he starts hearing about my vagina. Your Walnut stories and llama-drama brings us great joy.

And finally, thank you to the main man in my life who is always there for me and whose handsome good looks and strong character make me smile when I get up in the morning: Bertie. Without my little Bertie and Bonnie by my side, I'm not sure how many mornings I would've made it out of bed. Even though you're the most high maintenance dogs I could have asked for, my love for you is etched deep into my soul.

And finally – for real this time – thank you to the *real* main man in my life, who has been my partner, lover, friend, soul-mate, carpenter and comforter, not just over these

7 years but since the very first time I met you at Home Farm with Picasso. Ade, I know we may not have planned to be where we are right now, but I can honestly say there is no-one I would rather walk down this path with more than you. Thank you for loving me and our girls unconditionally like you do.

Extra Reading

Please take the time to do your own research on anything you've read in this book. Whilst there are literally hundreds of thousands of articles you could read on menopause, I have signposted you to a few here that you might find useful. Please also have a look at the websites of the specialists I've mentioned in the Acknowledgements section; their knowledge is invaluable.

Some suggested reading:

http://menopausesupport.co.uk

http://www.jodivine.com

https://www.harbornephysio.co.uk

https://menopausedoctor.co.uk

http://www.amandatozer.com

Useful search engine phrases to help find relevant information:

Please note: The following articles were relevant at the time of print but may be subject to availability in the future.

Womens health concern: "WHC factsheet HRT The history"

British Journal of Family Medicine: "BJFM vaginal dryness"

GSM Guidelines

GSM Top tips

Case Management Vaginal dryness

Thousands of women stopped having sex

Nice guidelines qs143

HRT hormone replacement therapy won't kill you but

ourworldindata record female life expectancy

Changing life expectancy ncbi pmc2625386

Oestrogen replacement article 44 4 551 67014